Metamorphosis in Care

D1566282

DEMENTIA
Metamorphosis in Care

CLAIRE BIERNACKI

Day Services Manager
Older People's Services
Derbyshire Mental Health Services NHS Trust

John Wiley & Sons, Ltd

55.00

Library of Congress Cataloging-in-Publication Data

Biernacki, Claire.
    Dementia : metamorphosis in care / by Claire Biernacki.
        p. ; cm.
    Includes bibliographical references and index.
    ISBN-13: 978-0-470-01997-9 (pbk.: alk. paper)
1. Dementia.   I. Title.
    [DNLM: 1. Dementia.   2. Dementia – nursing.   WM 220 B588d 2007]
    RC521.B54 2007
    616.8'3 – dc22

                                                2006032098

A catalogue record for this book is available from the British Library

ISBN-13: 978-0-470-01997-9

Typeset by TechBooks, Delhi, India.
Printed and bound in Great Britain by TJ International Ltd, Padstow, Cornwall.

This book is printed on acid-free paper responsibly manufactured from sustainable forestry in which at
least two trees are planted for each one used for paper production.

Dedication

I would like to thank Ruth, Caitlin and Sophie for their patience, support and encouragement throughout the completion of this book and express gratitude to those whose feedback and advice have been invaluable, in particular Sue O'Dea and Petrina Brown. I would also like to thank all those who have contributed to my education, in particular Jack, Olive, John, Phyllis, Mona, Kath and many, many others.

Contents

Preface

The past 20 years have seen an explosion of research and anecdotal evidence which calls into question virtually everything previously presented as fact with regard to the experience of dementia and people who have dementia. In 1997, the publication of the late Professor Kitwood's seminal work *Dementia Reconsidered* seemed to galvanise the activity, not only of academics but also of front line practitioners in seeking to re-define the meaning of care for persons with dementia. The term 'Person Centred Care' has become synonymous with this movement toward improving dementia care.

In the decade following Kitwood's publication, research has investigated aspects of dementia that would have been considered ridiculous 20 years ago, particularly aspects concerning the psychosocial elements of dementia and the subjective experience of dementia. As the evidence mounts, what is repeatedly confirmed is that there is a desperate and urgent need to alter care practices. Unfortunately what is also evident is that in reality little, if any, tangible change has occurred, despite this wealth of evidence. Persons with dementia still routinely find themselves in situations where their needs are secondary to those of others, where their value as individuals and indeed as human beings is denied. As someone who has worked in dementia care for 20 years, I have experienced the excitement that the arrival of 'Person Centred Care' generated and the disappointment that, at the point of delivery, care services seem barely to have registered a ripple of positive change. The personal frustration of this continuing situation led me to seriously consider leaving dementia care altogether. Instead I wrote this book.

This book takes the reader on a journey beginning with the history of dementia care, through the maze of ever increasing evidence into areas where positive change is taking hold and where cause for optimism is high; and into dark areas where people with dementia are emotionally abandoned and a sense of futility prevails.

The book uncovers the evidence for positive dementia care in a way that enables practitioners to understand why change is necessary, reinforcing the importance of theory to practice and detailing the skills practitioners need to acquire, in order to become expert practitioners in the dementia care specialism.

What this book will show is that approaches to positively influence the experience of dementia are readily available and clearly achievable. More than that, this book will show that adopting evidence-based approaches to care will improve the work satisfaction of practitioners. The book leaves practitioners at a crossroads, at a point in the evolution of the dementia care specialism, where choices have to be made with regard to how practice develops. Do we continue as we have been, digesting the evidence and changing the language of care but not really impacting on the quality of life of individuals in our care? Or do we accept that responsibility for initiating and supporting positive change belongs to each one of us who has chosen to spend their working lives caring for persons who have dementia? My sincere hope is that this book fosters a desire to adopt the latter approach.

1 Dementia in Context

INTRODUCTION

Chapter 1 provides an overview of dementia in the context of today's society, looking at what dementia is, the differential diagnoses and describing the main types of dementia together with some of the less common presentations, such as dementia in people with learning difficulties and in people of working age. This chapter considers how predicted changes in population are likely to impact on society and those living with dementia and considers dementia care from an historical perspective. The stigmatisation of people with mental health needs, including people with dementia, is a fact of our society that research finds to have altered little despite a move of care of these people into the community; this is described also in this chapter.

Many recently published texts on the care of the person with dementia deliberately avoid a definition and detailed description of signs, symptoms and types of dementia. This is understandable in an effort to de-medicalise care and to encourage the carer to look beyond the medical model, which is often seen as the antithesis of new models of care that encompass a person centred approach. I am including such a definition and description here for several reasons.

Firstly, throughout my years of clinical practice I have frequently witnessed carers accuse people with dementia of misbehaving, acting up and pretending they are unable to do something they could do only yesterday, and responding to this perceived misbehaviour with anger, and indeed punishment. This section of the book is about enabling carers to understand that the way in which the person with dementia behaves or communicates is directly affected by the damage that disease has caused to their brain. It is not behaviour designed to frustrate or anger the carer and responding to the behaviour with anger and admonishment is more than unhelpful; it is tantamount to abuse. It is now known that such a response on the part of carers is likely to result in much of the behaviour termed 'challenging' that people with dementia are labelled with. Interactions stemming from anger on the part of the carer have no place in the development of what is becoming the specialism of dementia care.

Secondly, knowledge of an individual's specific diagnosis, where it can be established, is vital in ensuring that correct information and advice are offered in a timely manner; for example, how the illness is likely to progress, what treatments are available, the likelihood of the disease being passed to children and other information the individual may seek.

Finally, while current evidence supports the view that interpersonal care based on a person centred model is the approach most likely to improve the quality of day-to-day life for the person with dementia, it is medical science that will provide the cure as it has begun to provide treatments. Just as we need to discard aspects of the medical care model that are detrimental to the individual's well-being so we need to take care that we maintain awareness of medical developments that will enhance our practice.

WHAT IS DEMENTIA?

There are surely more definitions of dementia than there are forms of dementia (approximately one hundred), so giving a definitive description is difficult. However, the World Health Organisation (1992) seems to encompass aspects that most agree on when it describes dementia as:

> A syndrome due to disease of the brain, usually of a chronic or progressive nature, in which there is impairment of multiple higher cortical functions, including memory, think- ing, orientation, comprehension, calculation, learning capacity, language and judgment. Consciousness is not clouded. The cognitive impairments are commonly accompanied, and occasionally preceded, by deterioration in emotional control, social behaviour, or motivation.

Thus this impairment has repercussions for the ability of people to manage aspects of their daily lives to their previous standard or ability. Tasks taken for granted such as washing, dressing, carrying on with work, hobbies and relationships become in- creasingly difficult. If the person lives long enough with dementia it may well become impossible for him or her to undertake these tasks independently or to communicate needs in easily understood ways.

The process of dementia is that it is a progressive syndrome; symptoms become more marked and impact more and more on the individual's life, eventually pervading all areas. For the purposes of loosely describing this process, different stages can be identified and are described in Tables 1.1 to 1.3. Consideration is given to the effects of dementia on cognitive function and the impact on behaviour and the emotions the individual may express as a result of the experience of dementia. This categorising is not intended nor should it be used as a means of labelling individuals who have dementia. It is incorrect to assume that any individual will have all of the symptoms or experiences described in the order described, because of course it is not only the process of disease and accompanying dementia that must be taken into account. We must also consider that person's personality, life history, physical state and social relationships.

WHAT IS NOT DEMENTIA?

Most diseases causing dementia are at present incurable, for example Alzheimer's disease, vascular disease and Lewy body disease. However, there are causes of

Table 1.1. Early stage dementia

Cognitive symptoms	Behaviour	Emotional response
Mild impairment of short term memory Difficulty with language and reading Difficulty making decisions Difficulty concentrating Difficulty making judgements Hallucinations (rare)	Forgetting birthdays, anniversaries, appointments Losing things Getting lost while driving Forgetting peoples' names Looking to others to confirm correctness of words or actions or conversely rejecting assistance offered Confabulating – making up information in the absence of the ability to recall correct information	Worry Social embarrassment Fear of going mad Suspicion Anxiety Denial Frustration Irritability Depression Tearfulness Unconcern

Table 1.2. Middle stage dementia

Cognitive symptoms	Behaviour	Emotional response
Loss of short term memory Patchy long term recall Dysphasia Difficulty planning, sequencing and using judgement Disorientation to time, place or person	Unable to pursue hobbies Unable to drive safely Misidentifying family members Loss of friendships and social contacts Disturbed sleep Difficulty with daily activities – washing, dressing, preparing food, shopping Walking and getting lost Self-harm attempt (rare)	Withdrawal Depression Paranoia Agitation/anxiety Apathy Anger Frustration Incongruence/lability Aggression Bereavement reaction Acceptance Tearfulness Unconcern

Table 1.3. Late stage dementia

Cognitive symptoms	Behaviour	Emotional response
Loss of short and long term memory Loss of judgment, planning and sequencing skills Severe dysphasia or aphasia Dysphagia Loss of ability to respond to own needs or express needs in easily understood ways	Unable to anticipate or meet daily needs – washing, dressing Incontinence Constant walking Difficulty with eating, drinking and self-feeding Social withdrawal Rejection of assistance – violence Repetitive actions and words/sounds	Placidity Agitation Anger Aggression Anxiety and panic Depression Complete withdrawal from interaction with others

dementia or more specifically conditions that appear to mimic dementia that are open to treatment. These include nutritional deficiencies, particularly B12 and folate, alcohol or drug abuse (although prolonged abuse can lead to irreversible dementia), minor head injury, depression, brain tumours and infective disease. All of these conditions can result in symptoms that are associated with dementia. A close examination of the onset, progression, nature and consistency of symptoms may aid accurate diagnosis but misdiagnosis can occur.

In the 1970s it was optimistically proposed that anywhere between 10 and 40 % of dementias might be reversible. A recent updated meta-analysis undertaken by Clarfield (2003) puts that figure very much lower. Ensuring thorough investigation to rule out a treatable cause or to treat what is treatable, however, is vital. As Clarfield points out 'comorbidity should always be treated for its own sake and in the hope that cognitive decline may at least be delayed'. It is therefore important that we are able to recognise and identify conditions that present with symptoms similar to dementia syndrome to enable appropriate treatment to be provided and to avoid misdiagnosis. Depression is one differential diagnosis that needs serious and thorough investigation. Differentiating between dementia and depression can be extremely difficult. In cases where the individual has a history of depressive episodes this may more strongly indicate depression. Although it is unusual for a first time episode of depression to occur in people aged over 65 years (outside of bereavement) this should not be discounted. Differentiation is further complicated by the fact that depression can and often does present co-morbidly and there is increasing evidence that depression can be an early warning sign of dementia.

Symptoms seen in both depression and dementia include memory impairment, disturbances in patterns of sleep, loss of interest in things that have been previously enjoyed, poor motivation and slowed thought processes. The underlying reasons for these changes are different. In dementia the damage to the brain is the causative factor. For individuals with depression recent memory is impaired as the ability to pay attention to and concentrate on new information is adversely affected as a result of depression, making the task of storing new information difficult. A further complication for people with depression may be that they fear this memory loss *is* dementia, which adds to their depressive feelings. Working with people with this type of memory loss can be very effective; teaching memory techniques and improving levels of concentration may be enough to resolve the difficulty. For people with dementia this is not the case as impairment in ability to learn new techniques is usually prohibitive.

Disturbances in sleep behaviour can also occur in both depression and dementia, but people with depression may have difficulty falling to sleep or may wake very early, whereas individuals with dementia more commonly experience disturbance throughout the night, sometimes due to disorientation to time. Therefore investigating the nature of sleep disturbance is important.

Dissecting the strands of common symptoms in this manner can assist accurate diagnosis but it is vital to differentiate as depression can be successfully treated. Importantly where a definitive diagnosis cannot be made the depression should be treated whatever its origin is thought to be, as this will improve the life quality of the individual if they prove to have dementia and support resolution of a true depressive illness.

A more accurate diagnosis of other conditions that produce symptoms similar to dementia can be slightly easier. A full screen of the individual's physical condition will highlight infectious illness which can cause an acute confusional state. It is also the case that acute confusion, as the term implies, has a sudden onset. Symptoms found in dementia can present in a matter of hours or days as the infection progresses; such onset is atypical in dementia. Again it is important to realise that where dementia exists an acute confusion caused by infection can also develop and again treatment to improve life quality and resolve acute symptoms is essential.

Nutritional deficiencies and alcohol and substance misuse may also be highlighted through a full physical screen and by taking a thorough history. While treatment of the former can be relatively easy to achieve, the abuse of alcohol and drugs, particularly for prolonged periods, is notoriously difficult to overcome. There is, however, an opportunity for those working with younger people who abuse such substances to include advice on dementia as a consequence of long term abuse in the hope that such health promotion may have a role in reducing the incidence of drug and alcohol related dementia in the future.

Where any individual presents with symptoms that are suggestive of dementia an important first step in diagnosis is to rule out any causes of symptoms that are not dementia. The treatable causes of dementia-like symptoms are certainly more straightforward than approaching the treatment of dementia, but it should be remembered a that definite diagnosis of dementia does not preclude the individual from suffering further illness that can potentially exacerbate symptoms and that when this occurs treatment is required. Therefore a person with dementia who exhibits an acute exacerbation of symptoms should have a physical screen to identify a physical health need that may be responsive to treatment, and thus it may be possible to treat acute symptoms and promote optimum life quality.

Evidence for Practice

What Is and What Is Not Dementia

Dementia is a progressive syndrome caused by diseases of the brain

Symptoms include problems with thinking, impairment of memory, orientation, comprehension, calculation and learning capacity, language and judgement difficulties and changes in behaviour

The behaviour and communication of people with dementia are affected by the damage the brain experiences as a result of dementia

Knowledge of the individual's diagnosis enables us to provide timely and appropriate information

It is vital to differentiate between dementia and treatable causes of dementia-like symptoms

Treatable causes of dementia-like symptoms include depression, nutritional deficiency, head trauma and alcohol abuse

Accurate diagnosis and the treatment of what is treatable is vital

Individuals with dementia may suffer from depression, infection or other illness that can exacerbate their symptoms, any change in behaviour requires investigation to rule out or treat these illnesses

ALZHEIMER'S DISEASE

Alzheimer's disease (AD) accounts for between 50 and 70 % of all dementias. It was first described by Alois Alzheimer in 1907. His case study portrayed the symptoms of a 51-year-old woman with a five-year history including the inability to care for herself and rejection of help, disorientation, failing memory and difficulty reading and writing. There was a gradual increase in severity of the symptoms and hallucinations also developed. The second case Alzheimer described was that of a 56-year-old man. Possibly as a result of Alzheimer's two cases AD was initially considered a rare form of pre-senile dementia.

In normal functioning the brain has two types of brain cell: the neuron and glial cell. Neurons are responsible for processing information and ensuring the brain works; glials protect and support neurons. Simply put, neurons form complex connections to complete brain tasks such as memory and language. Communication between neurons takes place at junctions termed synapses. Synapses pass information via chemical signals called neurotransmitters. Increased loss of one of these neurotransmitters, acetylcholine, is strongly associated with severity of AD. The damage caused by the disease process results in the brain becoming increasingly ineffective at passing messages essential for language, controlling movement and solving problems.

Why these changes happen and why some people but not others develop AD is not yet understood. It is thought probable that a combination of genetic propensity and biochemical, environmental and immune processes, all of which are being investigated, may prove to have a part to play. A very small number of people will inherit AD genetically, where a parent has the mutated gene a child will have a 50 % chance of developing the disease. Onset of the disease in this instance is generally between the ages of 40 and 50. As with all genetically inherited diseases it is important that those at risk are given the opportunity of counselling to enable them to make informed life choices, including whether or not to have children, to consider how to plan for the possible eventuality of their own ill-health and to support them in living with the prospect of developing such a life changing disease.

AD generally has a slow onset. Initially people may encounter difficulty recalling recent events, people's names, telephone numbers or where they put things. Memories from childhood or early adult life are usually recalled with little trouble. This can be puzzling as logic might suggest that what happened yesterday should be fresher in the mind than what happened when you were, for example, six years old. Although this memory difficulty may cause some concern it is often put down to the process of growing old. Health promotion that encourages people with memory difficulties to seek advice early will enhance the possibility of early diagnosis and treatment and provide reassurance where there is no cause for concern.

As the disease progresses symptoms of dementia become more pronounced, word finding difficulties become more common and memory impairment more serious. Appointments may be missed, medication overlooked and minor accidents can occur. At this stage it is difficult to rationalise what is happening as part of the ageing process.

At present there is no cure for AD but there are drugs that are licensed and were initially recommended by the National Institute for Clinical Excellence (2001) for the treatment of mild and moderate AD in the UK. These drugs, known by the group name acetylcholinesterase inhibitors, include donepzil, rivastigmine and galantamine and are discussed further in Chapters 2 and 8. While these drugs do not represent a cure for AD they do represent hope, a commodity in such short supply in dementia care that it has limited development of the specialty and consigned people with dementia to a bleak future. The hope presented is the hope that something rather than nothing can be done about this disease and the hope that the advancement of such drugs is the first step on a speedy journey to realistic cure or treatment to reverse the course of the disease.

Evidence for Practice

Alzheimer's Disease

AD accounts for 50–70 % of all cases of dementia

Seeking early diagnosis is advisable

Drug treatments in the form of acetylcholinesterase inhibitors are the first line treatment recommended for use in AD

In a minority of cases AD can be genetically inherited

Genetic counselling must be available for individuals where genetic inheritance is a possibility

---

VASCULAR DEMENTIA

There is disagreement in the literature as to whether vascular dementia is the second or third most common cause of dementia. Some experts suggest it may indeed be the most common in people over the age of 85. However, vascular dementia accounts for approximately 20 to 25 % of all dementias. The Alzheimer's Society (www.alzheimers.org.uk) reports that of the 750,000 people in the UK living with dementia one-quarter has vascular dementia.

Vascular dementia occurs when the blood supply to parts of the brain is restricted or blocked and the brain is deprived of oxygen; cells in the brain then die and symptoms of dementia result. Stroke or a series of strokes are common causes of vascular dementia. Indeed, stroke increases the risk of dementia by more than ninefold. A series of ministrokes leading to an accumulation of brain cell death and symptoms of dementia is termed multi-infarct dementia.

The risk factors for vascular dementia are similar to those for stroke disease and include hypertension, raised blood lipids, diabetes mellitus and smoking. As each of these risk factors is, for many people, linked to lifestyle choices, health promotion for the younger generation may impact on future numbers developing vascular dementia. Equally, the ability of medical science to treat stroke early may mean that greater numbers of people survive strokes but will live with stroke related dementia.

While education on risk factors may help reduce future numbers of sufferers it may also be possible to reduce the risk of further damage or multiple infarcts in those with an existing condition by advising and enabling them to choose healthier lifestyle options. Treatment with antihypertensives to control blood pressure and statins to lower blood lipids may also play a role. Amar and Wilcock (1996) report that 'evidence exists that controlling vascular risks such as hypertension and diabetes and using an antiplatelet drug can improve cognitive functioning'. Thus encouraging people with vascular disease to stop smoking and reduce fat in their diet and take prescribed drug treatments can have a positive impact on the progress of vascular dementia.

Evidence for Practice

Vascular Dementia

Vascular dementia accounts for at least 20 % of all dementias

Vascular dementia results from restricted blood flow to the brain and risk factors are similar to those for stroke disease

Offering health promotion advice on diet, alcohol consumption and smoking may reduce the risk of younger people developing vascular dementia

Choice of healthier lifestyle options by someone with existing vascular dementia may reduce the risk of progression of dementia

Although there is currently no treatment for vascular dementia, treatment to reduce risk of further vascular damage such as antiplatelets, antihypertensives and statins may help

Further strokes or ministrokes (transient ischaemic attacks) can occur and may result in further impairment

LEWY BODY DISEASE

Lewy body disease (LBD), also referred to as Lewy body dementia, diffuse Lewy body disease or senile dementia of Lewy body type, is characterised by fluctuating levels of alertness and cognition, hallucinations (most commonly visual), Parkinson's symptoms and the presence of dementia symptoms. LBD shares characteristics with both AD and Parkinson's disease and this can make accurate diagnosis difficult. The Parkinsonian symptoms commonly experienced are shuffling gait and falls. Fluctuation in ability, particularly cognitive ability, is not unusual in dementia, but with LBD this fluctuation can be from hour to hour and the difference between the best performance ability and the worst is more marked than in other dementias. It is vital that carers acknowledge this fluctuating ability and respond appropriately. For example, a person who was able to wash and dress independently in the morning may not be able to undress and get ready for bed in the evening; this is a result of the person having LBD not because he is awkward or seeking to annoy the carer by feigning inability or through laziness.

Temporary disturbances in consciousness are a feature of LBD, where the individual may be unresponsive for several minutes; such episodes can be confused with transient ischaemic attacks. Hallucinations often take the form of people or animals and can obviously be very distressing. One of the more difficult aspects of treatment of such psychotic symptoms is that the first choice of treatment in most other conditions, neuroleptic medication, has been found to be unsafe for people with LBD. There have been severe sensitivity reactions reported including increased drowsiness and impairment of consciousness and Keith (2002) reports a two- to threefold increase in mortality. On a more positive note Keith (2002) also reports that acetylcholinesterase inhibitors (the first line of treatment in Alzheimer's disease) elicit improvement in LBD and while they are not currently licensed for use in LBD they may soon become the first line of treatment.

Evidence for Practice

Lewy Body Dementia

People with Lewy body dementia experience gross fluctuations, often on a daily or even hourly basis, of cognition and functional ability

People with LBD experience symptoms associated with Parkinson's disease and are prone to falls

Hallucinations are common in the experience of someone who has LBD, which can be very distressing

Neuroleptic medication, often used to treat hallucinations, can be harmful when used as treatment in people with LBD

Acetylcholinesterase inhibitors may become the recommended treatment for LBD

FRONTOTEMPORAL DEMENTIA

Although not a common cause of dementia, frontotemporal dementia is worthy of discussion as the presentation can differ dramatically from what might be considered a typical presentation of dementia. Frontotemporal dementia is also thought to account for at least 20 % of all pre-senile dementias, having an onset between the ages of 40 and 65. It is the second most frequent cause of working-age dementia after AD, and family history is often found.

Personality, behaviour and reasoning are among the elements controlled by the brain's frontal and temporal lobes. Where a disease process or injury damages this area of the brain dramatic change in social behaviour and loss of personal awareness are evident. Normal social inhibitions are not effectively controlled and the person may become aggressive, withdrawn and stubborn, and not open to change. Sexual disinhibition may also be a feature and the person may fail to show appropriate emotional response to situations. Typically in the early stages memory is not impaired.

The behaviour of the person may be perceived as rude and intractable. The individual may also neglect personal hygiene and grooming needs. This has the potential to adversely affect the carer's regard for and inclusion of the individual and inflexible behaviour could be interpreted as a deliberate attempt to thwart the carer's efforts of help. The carer may struggle to reconcile apparent reasonable memory ability with evident reluctance to behave in a socially appropriate manner. Carers need to understand that damage to specific brain functions results in specific types of behaviour so that their expectations of the person's ability can be based on empathy rather than reprimand and on searching for skills that help the individual and allow for what might otherwise be considered unreasonable behaviour.

Evidence for Practice

Frontotemporal Dementia

Frontotemporal dementia is the second most common cause of working-age dementia

Onset is generally between the ages of 40 and 65

Dramatic changes in personality and social behaviour are features

Stubborn and resistive behaviour should be recognised as the result of dementia syndrome and not experienced as a personal affront by carers

Memory is not initially impaired

DEMENTIA AND PEOPLE WITH LEARNING DIFFICULTIES

People with learning difficulties have a higher incidence of developing dementia. This is particularly evident in people with Down's syndrome (DS) who are at greater risk of developing Alzheimer's disease (AD). Holland *et al.* (1998) found that prevalence rates for people with DS and AD were similar but occurred in people with DS 30 to 40 years earlier. By the age of 60 as many as 36 % of those with DS will have developed AD and by the age of 70 this will have risen to 54 %.

Given such prevalence of dementia in people with learning difficulties, it is clear that the need for accurate and early diagnosis is vital. However, diagnosing dementia in people with learning difficulties presents specific problems. Employing the commonly used cognitive screening tool, the mini mental state examination (Folstein *et al.* 1975) is inadequate given pre-existing cognitive impairment. Presentation of dementia may be both complex and atypical in people with DS. Stanton and Coetzee (2004) discuss the many difficulties that may be encountered in trying to achieve correct diagnosis, including changes in behaviour being attributed to the existing learning disability rather than dementia and difficulty in establishing subjective symptoms because of poor communication and social skills. Where such complexity exists in establishing a diagnosis, compiling as full a history as possible in order that current behaviour and functioning can be compared with historical behaviour and functional ability is called for.

Caring for people with learning difficulties who have dementia is complicated by poor tolerance of drug treatments, and while Stanton and Coetzee point out that acetylcholinesterase inhibitors may be used there is little in the way of research evidence to confirm their effectiveness. This is unlikely to alter in the near future as a label of learning difficulties generally excludes individuals from inclusion in research trials.

Cooper and Prasher (1998) found that for people with learning difficulties and their carers behavioural symptoms can be of greater significance than the cognitive changes caused by dementia. They found that low mood, restlessness and excessive overactivity, a disturbed sleep pattern and uncooperative behaviour were more prevalent, as were auditory hallucinations in people with DS, while in people with intellectual disability other than DS, aggression occurred with greater frequency.

Fromage and Anglade (2002) highlight the fact that, given changes in life expectancy, an older generation of people with learning difficulties is a new group in society and as such the body of knowledge informing their care is meagre. A combination of what is known about people with learning difficulties and what is being learnt about presentation of dementia in this group should begin to inform practice. Stanton and Coetzee (2004) urge careful consideration of the environment in which the individual is cared for. They identify any change in the stability of the person's environment or those around them as a potential threat to well-being, which may contribute to an exacerbation of dementia. Conversely, moving to a new but more suitable environment sooner rather than later may be beneficial in allowing the individual to adapt before deterioration in cognitive function makes this more difficult. This conundrum is familiar to many of us working with other people with dementia and indeed a sharing of skills and knowledge between carers of people with learning difficulties and carers of people with dementia will benefit recipients of care. For example, for people with DS it is no less important to identify the cause of dementia and to treat what can be treated. Coetzee and Stanton conclude that the aim of care is to slow the progress of decline and encourage adaptation, attend to distress and relieve symptoms. This is no less appropriate for those with dementia with no learning difficulties as for those with a learning difficulty who develop dementia.

Evidence for Practice

Dementia and People with Learning Difficulties

People with learning difficulties, particularly Down's syndrome, have an increased likelihood of developing dementia, particularly AD

Accurate diagnosis of dementia in people with learning difficulties is very difficult

People with learning difficulties are particularly prone to the side effects of medication

Careful consideration should be given to the timing and appropriateness of any change in environment

A sharing of knowledge between dementia care workers and those working with people with learning difficulties should benefit both specialisms

---

WORKING-AGE DEMENTIA

This term is used to describe dementia when it occurs in people under the age of 65; the terms early onset dementia and pre-senile dementia are also used. Although not a common disease in this age group, there is still a significant number of people in the UK who are affected by dementia at a younger age. The Alzheimer's Society website provides figures of one in 1000 people between the ages of 40 and 65 living with dementia.

Diagnosing dementia in this age group is difficult and specialist services to meet the specific needs of younger people are sparse throughout the country. However, given the pervasive and progressive nature of dementia, special consideration and services are vital in meeting the needs of those who develop and have to live with dementia at a younger age. Dementia at any age is a devastating diagnosis and while it would be patronising to hold that it matters slightly less to develop it when you are 'old', it should be acknowledged that younger people might have quite different needs.

Personal, family and career expectations for the future become undermined by the diagnosis. Those who are in employment and in many cases the family breadwinner, with dependent children and significant financial commitments, may find it even harder to come to terms with losing the abilities and skills required to continue their family role. Contemplating the prospect of being cared for rather than being carer within the family milieu brings considerable emotional stress.

Even where younger people are able to access services established for older people few services are geared for meeting such disparate emotional and practical needs as those faced by people who are 40 and those who are 90, together with the generations between. The outcome may well be that the younger person disengages from services, thus putting further strain on the home situation and increasing their feelings of being a burden.

The solution lies in providing specific services for people with working-age dementia. Services should provide early diagnosis and recognise and respond to the disruption of emotional, psychological, financial and family life that dementia can elicit. Few such services currently exist and as dementia care is an area that finds it difficult to attract health service funding for the majority it is unlikely that any new money will be forthcoming to develop a specific resource nationally for the minority with working-age dementia. This should not deter us from demanding further funds and supporting campaigns such as the Alzheimer's Society campaign in demanding these services. Nor should it prevent us from using existing money imaginatively or seeking other ways of changing existing services to suit younger people. The emotional impact of the experience of dementia for individuals younger than 65 is discussed further in Chapter 5.

Evidence for Practice

Working-Age Dementia

One in 1000 people between the age of 40 and 65 have dementia

The experience of dementia at a younger age imposes different needs

Specific areas of need include employment, family relationships and role, finance and psychological support

Few services are available to meet the needs of this minority group

Those providing services need to campaign for more funds, but to also be imaginative in using existing funding and services to address shortfalls in the service

---

DEMOGRAPHY, STATISTICS AND THEIR IMPLICATIONS

Dementia is primarily, though not exclusively, a disease of older age. While one in 1000 people under the age of 65 will have dementia, one in 20 people over 65 years will be affected, rising to one in five after the age of 80. Life expectancy rates have altered dramatically over the past one hundred years. In 1901 the life expectancy for women was 49 years and for men 41, meaning that dementia was relatively rare. According to the National Statistics Office's website (www.statistics.gov.uk), life expectancy for women in 2002 was 84 years and for men 81 years. With this increase in life expectancy comes an increased likelihood of developing dementia.

Dementia has been found to occur in every country in the world. It is estimated that 18 million people worldwide have dementia and that this figure will almost double to 34 million by 2025. In the United Kingdom the estimate by 2050 is that some 1.8 million people will be living with dementia. This is causing considerable concern. This dramatic rise in life expectancy has been accompanied by a fall in birth rates, prompting speculation of demographic time-bombs where a rapidly ageing society will be unsustainable by a dwindling working-age population.

Indeed, with figures provided by the National Statistics Office of 74 % of women and 67 % of men living with long term illness or disability over the age of 85, it is easy to conclude that the problems associated with growth in an ageing population may overwhelm existing resources for health and social care. In Australia, for example, there is much talk of a dementia epidemic, with the largest source of disability burden expected to be dementia by 2016, and where between 1995 and 2041 the number of people with dementia is expected to increase by 254 %, while the total population increases by 40 %. There has been some criticism of viewing dementia and people with dementia in such negative terms as a source of 'disability burden', but with projected statistics indicating rises in the old age population and accompanying concern about low birth rates in the developed world it may be difficult to avoid negative overtones.

The Alzheimer's Society (2006) takes a more positive view, stressing that the rate of growth will be gradual and that as long as appropriate resources are developed and financed then as Coleman (2001) suggests in this country 'demographic time bombs only go off in the media, not in real life'.

Many leading organisations concur that the development of strategies in line with predicted changes in population are vital. These include calls for more research into the causes, cure and treatment of dementia, the development of strategies to meet the needs of people with dementia at both local and national level, early diagnosis and treatment of dementia with support following diagnosis and support for carers and the caring relationship.

That dementia is becoming a national health priority is clear in the minds of those working with people who have dementia, but what is needed now is to alert the general public and local and national government to the issues. Again organisations like the Alzheimer's Society and Alzheimer Scotland are in the forefront of such action. The difficulties in achieving success are numerous, not least the fact that many 'epidemics' can be seen to be vying for government attention and funding – drugs, alcohol, teenage pregnancies and terrorism to cite but a few. However, these difficulties should not detract from the efforts made in pursuing improvements and securing resources to benefit the lives of those affected by dementia.

A BRIEF HISTORY OF DEMENTIA CARE

The Oxford English Dictionary at the end of the eighteenth century defines dementia as coming from the Latin *demens* and meaning 'senseless, mad, foolish'. An earlier description given by Cosin in 1592 (from Hunter & Macalpine 1963) defines dementia as: 'A passion of the mind, bereaving it of the light of understanding. When a man's perceivance and understanding of all things is taken away'. The availability of such definitions demonstrates the historical recognition of dementia and enables understanding of why people with dementia came to be placed in the large workhouses and asylums of the 1800s and why dementia care became inexorably linked with care of the mentally ill.

An extract from the 1844 Report of the Metropolitan Commissioners in Lunacy, which sought to define various forms of insanity, characterises dementia as 'the decay and obliteration of intellectual faculties'. Along with mania it was the prevailing form of insanity afflicting inhabitants of the large institutions that protected society from the lunatics into the twentieth century. Therefore, not only has there long been a recognisable definition and some understanding of the effects of dementia it has for many years accounted for a large proportion of places allocated for people with mental health problems.

Three distinct periods have been identified by Thornicroft and Tansella (2003) in the development of mental health care. Firstly, the rise of the asylum period between 1880 and 1950, secondly, the decline of the asylum beginning in the 1950s and, finally, balanced care, which can be identified as currently being underway. By all accounts the asylums were places of containment, where chains and manacles and the provision of the bare essentials of food and shelter were the method of treatment. While society as a whole may have been seen to gain protection from this system it could hardly be described as a caring approach to people with mental health problems, people with dementia included. As Rollin (2003) identifies, the asylums were in effect society's dustbins, where as well as bona fide patients staff had to deal with:

> An assorted rag-bag of social misfits: people with varying grades of learning disability; those addicted to drugs and alcohol, either acutely or chronically disturbed; those with personality disorders of protean varieties; vagrants; the aged who had become an embarrassment to their kin; pregnant single women who had been cast out by their relatives; and anyone who by hook – and not infrequently by crook – could be squeezed into whatever the law required to be certified.

The decline of the asylum period is described as a time of recognition of the ill-effects of the asylum system. Thornicroft and Tansella (2003) list the many shortcomings of the asylum system, including the ill-treatment of patients and the effects of institutionalism. The decline of the asylum system is characterised by prevention of admissions through provision of community facilities, discharging of institutionalised patients and the establishment and maintenance of community support systems. It is interesting to note that as asylums closed and are closing the last inhabitants to leave are not infrequently those patients with dementia. This perhaps indicates a lack of awareness of how to prepare the community to care for people with dementia and reluctance to provide the resources required to successfully meet the needs of people with dementia outside the asylum.

By the 1960s a more sympathetic approach to the treatment of the mentally ill was emerging and various psychological therapies were among the accepted treatments. However, psychological therapies for older people and in particular for people with dementia were slow in developing. This can be accounted for by continued ageism and the low professional status attached to working with older people. The elderly also suffered from the stereotype of being untreatable, a view propounded by Freud (1905) himself, who considered those over fifty years of age to be 'ineducable'. Indeed, historically psychotherapy has little in the way of theory to underpin the development of therapies for older people. In an overview of psychotherapies with older people Hepple (2004) identifies that only Erikson acknowledges the developmental challenges of later life and the paucity of development of his work or any further contributions on theories of old age has left psychotherapy for older people not only detached from mainstream psychotherapy but without a theoretical base.

The nursing profession also had little to offer in developing care or therapies for people with dementia before the 1980s. Indeed, many of the earlier nursing texts served only to reinforce negative images of the elderly and in particular people with dementia and to strengthen accepted opinion that where there was no cure there was no hope. Information taken from nursing literature of the time exemplifies this clearly. The Nurses Aid series of books was one of the most popular sources of nursing knowledge and in 1977 authors Altschul and Simpson had the following cautions for care of the elderly: 'Old people are slower in their activities than are the young, and there are many things that they cannot do at all.' As examples they added that old people could not climb stairs, should never use a ladder, may be antagonistic and rebellious and find it tiring to raise their arms to comb their hair! Fortunately, the authors go on to highlight 'there are now many aids for the disabled that can be adapted for the elderly'. With regard to dementia care Altschul and Simpson urged nurses to be 'concerned primarily with the preservation of physical health' and pointed out that 'a great deal of suffering can be spared to the patient and his relatives if his appearance is well preserved and he remains socially acceptable for the longest possible time'. While we would today not contradict this advice it would certainly not be considered our primary concern.

Despite the dearth in available treatments for people with dementia during the 1960s and 1970s one treatment did emerge which was claimed as a major advancement in the care of people with dementia; this was reality orientation (RO). For some 30 years RO was touted as the treatment of choice for those providing care for people with dementia. RO techniques are based on the repetitive presentation of information regarding time, place and person so that the person can relearn and retain this information. One of the difficulties that had been observed in people with dementia was that increasing disorientation led to social withdrawal, which resulted in a lack of sensory stimulation. The repeated information giving of RO was aimed at improving orientation, avoiding understimulation and sustaining interaction with others. This it was felt would improve self-esteem and reduce the risk of problem behaviour developing. The success of RO is dependent on everyone involved with the individual using the technique and employing both 24-hour orientation (as the term implies throughout the day, in each interaction) and in a more formal classroom situation where lessons in orientation are undertaken. RO can be delivered one to one or in group situations.

RO is still in use today; RO boards displaying the address, date and such pertinent information are a frequent sight in many institutional care settings. However, there is little to support its use and some evidence contradicts the claims that RO can improve self-esteem. One of the obvious flaws that quickly assails those using RO for the first time is that this repetition of information can actually serve to distress some individuals as they are repeatedly reminded that they cannot retain that most basic of information: day, date and where they are. For most people expressing distress and showing signs of disorientation the main concern is not whether it is Monday or Tuesday, August or December but how did I get here and when can I go home? Despite the many criticisms of RO it might be foolish to completely dismiss the technique, as with many therapies success is dependent on appropriate application. In a recent review of the evidence for classroom-based RO, Spector *et al.* (2000) found that there are benefits on both cognition and behaviour for people with dementia, although which features of RO brought about this improvement and whether or not it was sustainable at the end of treatment requires further research.

In the history of a developing dementia care specialism RO is important. Here was an approach that encouraged interaction with the person with dementia, something that was done *with* rather than *to* the individual. RO demands that carers interact directly with the person with dementia; it has been argued that in itself that is the real benefit of RO.

Hot on the heels of RO another interpersonal technique for use in dementia care was being developed by Feil (1982), termed validation therapy. Feil had experience of the advent of RO growing up with parents involved in dementia care who were exponents of the new therapy. She found that employing RO caused distress, particularly in very old people who had lived with dementia for some years. Feil's method can be seen as a humanistic approach based on accepting another's reality and experience rather than trying to insist they accept ours. Validation therapy can therefore be viewed as a person centred approach aimed at restoring dignity, engendering respect of the individual and concentrating on avoiding degeneration into a vegetative state. Use of empathy is the key to employing validation techniques. Feil's development of her own model, including describing stages of dementia and accompanying communication methods, has come in for some criticism as it was not developed from an accepted theoretical base and her classification of the stages of dementia does not replicate accepted medical systems.

A review of the effectiveness of validation therapy carried out by Neal and Briggs (2003) can only call for more research into this therapy, as existing studies are inconclusive. What is clear is that in terms of focusing the nurse–patient relationship on the experience of the patient in the 1980s Feil was ahead of her time and some commentators; among them Morton (1997) put Feil at the forefront of the focus on the *experience* of dementia.

STIGMA, DISCRIMINATION AND DEMENTIA

Consideration of stigma and discrimination in the fields of both mental illness and old age has been well researched and widely commented upon. With recent research into the experience of dementia we are beginning to gather and understand information about the effects of stigma that people with dementia experience. Unsurprisingly there is evidence that stigma leads to discrimination against people with dementia on the part of society as a whole, but perhaps a little more surprisingly discrimination on the part of the very people charged with funding, developing and delivering services for people with dementia is also evident. The very gatekeepers of services are themselves restricting services because they hold beliefs that old people and people who are mentally ill are less deserving of help than other sectors of society.

According to the World Health Organisation (2001), 'Stigma can be defined as a mark of shame, disgrace or disapproval which results in an individual being shunned or rejected by others.' Stigma erodes the premise that all people are created equal, depriving people of their dignity, denying their full participation in society and reducing their entitlement to the same rights as others. Common stereotypes held about people with a psychiatric diagnosis are identified throughout the literature and include that they are a danger to others, difficult to talk to, unpredictable, have only themselves to blame for their affliction, and need to pull themselves together. It is also widely held that people will never recover from mental illness and that treatment will not improve their condition (Crisp *et al.* 2000). Byrne (2000) describes the experience of stigma as causing the individual shame, blame, isolation and social exclusion. The resulting effects are multiple. People with mental health problems are reluctant to seek help, as being open about a psychiatric diagnosis is seen as inviting stigmatisation.

Stereotypes of old people are that they are a burden, sick, weak, vulnerable, intractable and largely responsible for their own misfortunes. People with dementia experience a double weight of stigma, as they are viewed as being both old and mentally ill. When people with dementia are of a different race, culture or sexual orientation the incidence of stigma and discrimination on multiple fronts can occur.

A Royal College of Psychiatrists Report (2001) into stigmatisation and discrimination within the medical profession found that doctors, psychiatrists included, give up on some patients with serious mental illness, relegating them to second-class status with regard to the health care system. Indeed, psychiatric services stand accused of contributing to misconceptions about mental illness (Byrne 2000). The Royal College of Psychiatrists in their campaign entitled *Changing Minds: Every Family in the Land* (2006) identify that, as medical practitioners are often the first port of call for people seeking support or treatment, it is crucial such assistance is not hampered by prejudice on the part of the very people who control access to appropriate services.

The detrimental and pervasive influence of stigma is beginning to be addressed. The recent Department of Health National Service Frameworks for Mental Health (1999) and Older Adults (2001) give priority to tackling the adverse effects of stigma. The frameworks lead respectively with standards designed to combat discrimination and promote social inclusion of individuals with mental health problems and to tackle age discrimination in order that it becomes a thing of the past. As carers of people with dementia, the onus is on us to consider our attitudes to both old people and people with mental health problems, to consider whether we, as the people who have chosen this field of practice, in fact believe that people with dementia are slightly less deserving of funding and services than younger, mentally fitter individuals. If people with dementia cannot rely on those of us who have *chosen* to work with them to do so in a nondiscriminatory way there may be little hope of real progress and positive change in care practices.

CONCLUSION

Already we are beginning to see that practising within the field of dementia care means developing understanding, knowledge and skills on many levels and in a multitude of areas. In this first chapter alone we have encountered seven variations of the syndrome and considered implications for practitioners. We have looked at other causes of dementia-like symptoms and the process of differentiation. We have seen how dementia care became aligned with mental health care and the stagnation in development of psychotherapeutic approaches. We have raised an awareness of the role of stigma within care practices and the need to examine our own approach to care to ensure we do not perpetrate discrimination. In the 30 years since Altshul and Simpson advised against allowing old people to climb ladders some things have changed and people with dementia are less likely to inhabit large wards in the asylums, but what else has altered? This is the question this book will address. There is a growing evidence base from which to deliver care that should be influencing the role of people with dementia in society and within the context of the caring relationship. That evidence and whether or not this influence is apparent in real terms are considered throughout this book.

2 Impetus for Change

INTRODUCTION

During the past 20 years there have been significant developments in the way we, as a society and as carers, view persons with dementia and the experience of dementia. A growing base of evidence, both researched and anecdotal, is now available that should inform and guide our care approaches. That these advances have led to little in the way of real change to the benefit of people with dementia in various care environments will be keenly debated elsewhere in this book.

However, given the depth of information these developments bring there can be little doubt that we as carers and those with dementia are on the verge of tangible positive change. Ensuring that we exploit these developments to enlighten and improve care and the life quality of those living with dementia will require skilful change management and the translation of the evidence base into practice.

A good starting point is consideration of what has happened over the preceding 20 years that indicates the necessity for change. This chapter identifies the key drivers to the development of new theory bases and effective therapeutic approaches in caring for people with dementia.

Drivers for change have come from several directions. Consideration is given to the powerful outcomes achieved by those few well-known public figures that have chosen to be open and to share their diagnosis of dementia with the world in the hope of improving the lot of the millions around the world diagnosed with some form of dementia. Other bottom-up drivers for change are also discussed, including person centred care and challenges to the long held belief that people with dementia have no discernible experience, the significant growth in research based evidence about the experience of dementia, the influence of the Alzheimer's Society and the impact of developments in the pharmaceutical industry. Top-down drivers in the form of government policy and initiatives, including the Community Care Act (Department of Health 1990) and The National Service Framework for Older People (2001) and changes in nurse education, both in training and continuous development, can be seen to be having an influence on the way dementia care is developing.

These drivers have informed public and professional opinion and behaviour, challenged stigma and discrimination, and motivated calls for urgent and radical change in the way services are designed for people who have dementia. All of this is seeking to propel the concept of dementia services from a little acknowledged subsection of psychiatry, staffed by those not quite dynamic enough for other areas of psychiatry, to a forward thinking dynamic specialism – a specialism where people with dementia are considered the controlling partners in care and familial carers the experts.

BOTTOM-UP DRIVERS FOR CHANGE

FAME AND DEMENTIA

Given the incidence of dementia among the general population it is easy to understand that many well-known people must have succumbed to the effects of the condition: film stars, literary figures, politicians, sports personalities and leaders of industry. Dementia is no respecter of reputation, intelligence or worldly status. Among those thought, or known, to have had dementia are actress Margaret Rutherford, boxer Sugar Ray Robinson, authors Somerset Maugham, Enid Blyton and Iris Murdoch, politicians Harold Wilson and Ronald Reagan, artist Norman Rockwell, Princess Juliana of the Netherlands and actors Charles Bronson, Rita Hayworth and Charlton Heston. This list is not intended to be sensationalist but to enable us to consider that stigma leads many people to hide their diagnosis and also to reflect on the hugely beneficial influence those who are open about their diagnosis have brought to a developing specialism.

The stigma attached to having dementia and the widespread discrimination against people with dementia cannot be underestimated. In a society where youthfulness and a quick brain are qualities to be admired those no longer youthful and with unreliable cognition feel their uselessness keenly. We have already seen the effect of stigma in relation to mental health and considered that even within the field of mental health care older people are further discriminated against by virtue of their age.

In the light of this it is perhaps easy to understand why many famous figures have been reluctant to disclose a diagnosis of dementia in themselves or family members. Fame and often fortune are closely linked in our society to positive media representation; where people perceive themselves as shameful, self-image is negative and portrayal of this in the media is perceived as leading to only negative outcomes. However, this has not proven to be the case. For those brave few who have been open about their diagnosis of dementia and the effects on their life the benefits to others with the syndrome and the benefits in raising the public profile, educating society and extending research has been powerful.

In 1994 the former actor and president of the United States, Ronald Reagan, revealed that he had been diagnosed with Alzheimer's disease. In an open letter to the American people Reagan (1994) explained that he hoped by sharing his diagnosis he would promote greater awareness of the condition and 'encourage clearer understanding of the individuals and families who are affected by it'.

Following his death, Verdantam (2004), writing in *The Washington Post*, described the contribution Ronald Reagan and his wife have made to the cause, declaring that 'an Alzheimer's diagnosis means something very different today than when former president Ronald Reagan announced 10 years ago that he had the illness'. The article goes on to say that Reagan was personally responsible for dramatically reducing the stigma attached to dementia. In raising funds and challenging government positioning on research into embryonic stem cell research for Alzheimer's Nancy Reagan wielded, and continues to wield, the kind of authority most pressure groups hoping to influence the powers that be can only dream of.

In 1994 the Reagans set up the Ronald and Nancy Reagan Research Institute with the Alzheimer's Association of America to accelerate research into Alzheimer's disease. Their celebrity raised the public profile of dementia, making it more acceptable and less shameful to have the syndrome, and brought in donations estimated in millions. This money was used and continues to be used to fund numerous research projects searching for the treatment and cure of dementia.

Actor Charlton Heston revealed that he too had been diagnosed with symptoms consistent with Alzheimer's disease. In a videotaped announcement Heston (2002) explained: 'If you see a little less spring in my step, if your name fails to leap to my lips, you'll know why. And if I tell you a funny story for the second time, please, laugh anyway.' Heston also chose not to withdraw from public life completely or hide away. He joined forces with the Academy of Molecular Imaging in calling for increased use of positron emission tomography (PET) scans, for the early diagnosis of Alzheimer's disease. Having been diagnosed in the early stages of AD by PET scan he realised the importance of using the technology to enable early diagnosis in others so that available treatment could be sought as soon as possible. He realised also the power of attaching his name to promotion of the scan as a means of adding influence to the campaign for early diagnosis.

In Australia the ex-wife of former prime minister Bob Hawke has been praised for disclosing her own diagnosis of dementia. She, together with Alzheimer's Australia (www.alzheimers.org.au), has established the Hazel Hawke Alzheimer's Research and Care Fund. It is planned that the fund will use donations to provide services and support for people with dementia and their families, including counselling, website and library facilities, carer education, public awareness raising and advocacy on policy issues on behalf of people with dementia, as well as undertaking research. Few spokespeople from medical, research or nursing backgrounds could have the positive impact that such public disclosures by well-known people with dementia have. With high media access such figures enable greater understanding of dementia and its influence on lives, and in so doing they challenge the negative stereotypes that breed fear and shame and instead foster understanding and acceptance. Others living with the condition are enabled to feel normal, stand a little taller and empowered to speak out about their own situation as well as benefiting from the increased funds and research generated. The message portrayed is that dementia is not something that needs to be hidden but is something worthy of attention so that life quality for those with dementia can improve. The actions of these few well-recognised public figures have driven change in dementia care, from public perception to research into cure – change that is drastically needed.

RESEARCH IN DEMENTIA

The evidence base for dementia care and treatment has grown beyond all recognition in the past 20 years. Today there are few issues around dementia for which there is no research evidence to consult. Much of this research may be in its infancy compared to advances in other diseases and much of it may culminate in calls for further research, but much of it also provides new information about people with dementia and their needs that demands urgent and radical change to the ways in which we undertake our practice and support people with dementia. The vast majority of this research has focused on the psychosocial aspects of dementia, asking what happens to people who have dementia, what it feels like to have dementia, gathering information on the outcomes of particular interventions, trying to establish the best way to support carers, examining the physical environments that people with dementia are expected to live in or asking whether to disclose the diagnosis to people with dementia.

In their 2004 review Bamford *et al.* identified 59 studies aimed at gathering information about diagnosis disclosure. While their review suggests that the views of people with dementia are under-represented and not enough information is available to enable a definitive approach to disclosure to be described, the significant point for the world of dementia care must surely be the growth of study in this area. There can be little doubt that diagnosis disclosure to the person with dementia is a growing concern for carers, both professional and familial, but 20 years ago there was no concern; people with dementia were simply not told. This is a prime example of how research is demanding change in our practice.

Initially most research into psychosocial aspects of dementia concentrated on gaining information by proxy and carers' opinions were considered the best method of informing practice. Directly involving people with dementia in research has long been considered problematic, primarily due to issues around obtaining informed consent and perceived difficulties in communication. In very simple terms much research is dependent on asking questions, with the expectation that research subjects respond to the questions, with consensus among answers being considered evidence. The presumption that people with dementia would not be able to provide consistent answers to research questions excluded their involvement. However, two factors demand that we increasingly involve people with dementia in research: firstly, it is possible and they can answer questions and, secondly, it is only by consulting with people with dementia that we will be able to define, develop and evaluate services that specifically meet the needs of people with dementia. Indeed, research is beginning to reflect the problems of basing care approaches on the needs of proxy informants. In the area of diagnosis disclosure carers and most professionals, when asked, thought that people with dementia should not be given their diagnosis, but when people with dementia are asked the overwhelming majority want to know what is wrong with them.

Arguably the greatest impact on dementia care is the research undertaken to document the experience of dementia. What we learn from this research will enable us to change the quality of life for those living with the disease and those close to them and indeed to improve our own job satisfaction. Keady (1996) is critical of many studies for the small samples used to draw conclusions, but again they represent a significant move forward in trying to document what it is like to have dementia and the implications for practice are tangible. It is now not only acceptable but repeatedly demanded (Cotrell & Schulz 1993; Wilkinson 2002) that people with dementia are actively involved in research and that they are directly asked the questions we need answers to in order to inform practice.

It is no accident that journals specifically aimed at the dementia care market and dementia care professionals first began to appear in the 1990s (*The Journal of Dementia Care* first appeared in 1993, *Signpost* in 1997 and *Dementia: The International Journal of Social Research and Practice* in 2002) for it was in the 10 years prior to this that an interest in questioning through research the accepted knowledge about dementia began to galvanise. Such journals reflect the need to update practitioners at every level on the new information that research is providing in the care specialism so that changes to practice can be made.

Methods of research in dementia care have been criticised, sample groups are too small and the information gathered is too broad or is inconsistent, but surely the salient point is that research in dementia care is happening and it is increasingly involving people with dementia. To a certain extent it is frightening as well, because what the research is largely telling us is that the presumptions upon which we have based care approaches to date are false; research is a primary driver for change in dementia care.

THE ALZHEIMER'S SOCIETY

In 1979 when the then Alzheimer's Disease Society was established few people outside the medical profession had heard of Alzheimer's disease. In marking the Society's twenty-fifth anniversary the chairman, Dr Nicholas Carey, in the Alzheimer's Society's Annual Review (2004) reported that campaigning by the Society 'has influenced government debate and helped to bring about changes to the law', to the benefit of people living with dementia and those caring for them. Over its 25 year history the Society has grown from a two branch organisation to having 264 branches and support groups across England, Wales and Northern Ireland. The Society's aims have remained consistent: to increase awareness about dementia, to provide support, education and information for carers and to improve the quality of life and care that people with dementia experience. The Society also funds medical and scientific research.

Since its inception the Society has undertaken a phenomenal amount of activity in every area. Alzheimer's disease is a term now recognised readily by the man in the street. People with dementia, family carers, relatives and friends consistently express a sense of relief on contacting the Society and meeting people in similar circumstances, accessing the information they need from people who have been in the same situation and can advise first hand on the pitfalls and benefits of different courses of action. The Society provides over 80 fact sheets giving information on subjects ranging from types of dementia to brain tissue donation. The Society has achieved numerous milestones, all of which have led to an increased public awareness of the disease and brought about action to benefit people touched by dementia.

Among the campaigns championed by the Society are demands for free health care for people with dementia, access to antidementia drugs, high quality care standards, legislation to protect the rights of people with dementia to make decisions and a cessation of the overprescription of neuroleptic drugs for people with dementia. The 2004 Report identified that the Society made considerable contributions to improving life quality for people with dementia, sending a CD-ROM to every primary care practice manager in the United Kingdom (11,500 in all), contributing one million pounds to research into the cause, cure and care of dementia, operating a telephone helpline taking 20,000 calls a year and a website receiving 72,000 hits per month. By April 2004 the Society was also providing training for 300 care workers per month and the project 'Food for Thought' gave carers access to information aimed at improving the nutritional status of people with dementia. The influence of the activity of the Alzheimer's Society on care experiences and expectations of people who have dementia and their carers is significant and is likely to continue to be so. The impact of the activity of the Alzheimer's Society in this country and an international federation of 69 Alzheimer associations throughout the world under the umbrella of Alzheimer's Disease International (http://www.alz.co.uk/) has already proven important in achieving change in dementia care practices. By continuing to demand attention from government, raising issues important to people with dementia and their carers and campaigning for a better life for individuals with dementia and their carers the Society will undoubtedly persist in being a key driver of change in this area.

THE PHARMACEUTICAL INDUSTRY

In the late 1990s the first drugs for the treatment of Alzheimer's disease (AD) were licensed for use in the United Kingdom. The benefits of the arrival of treatment for AD have so far been measured in terms of effectiveness on the dementing condition. Issues considered include whether or not the progress of dementia is arrested, if so for how long and what benefits there are to a carer's stress levels or to an individual's behavioural abilities. These are subjects that have been investigated by research, the conclusions reached often proving to be contradictory. However, perhaps the most important outcome of the advent of treatment for AD is that it means that AD (and by default all dementias) is no longer a hopeless condition. Something can be done. These drug treatments offer something that has long been missing in dementia care; they offer hope. The power of this hope as the impetus and driver for change should not be underestimated.

The four drugs currently licensed for use in AD in the United Kingdom are donepzil (Aricept), rivastigmine (Exalon), galantamine (Reminyl) and memantine (Ebixa). The first three drugs are known as acetylcholinesterase inhibitors. In simple terms acetylcholine is a neurotransmitter important for memory function and is severely affected by AD. Acetylcholinesterase is an enzyme that destroys acetylcholine; these drugs block the action of the destructive enzyme, thus increasing the amount of acetylcholine available for memory function and slowing down the progress of AD. They are licensed for use with mild to moderate dementia and the guidelines dictate that they should be discontinued once effectiveness ceases, this being determined by the level of deterioration over a period of time. Their free availability on the National Health Service, determined by the National Institute for Health Excellence (NICE), was initially advised for those with mild to moderate Alzheimer's, but a review ongoing in 2006 looks likely to come to a decision that those with moderate Alzheimer's only will have free access to these drugs.

Memantine was first licensed in the United Kingdom in 2002 and is indicated for treatment for those in the later stages of AD. The action of memantine is different in that it claims to treat symptoms rather than halt disease progress. Memantine works on the N-methyl-D-aspartate receptors (NMDA) in the brain, preventing calcium build-up that can further damage cells already damaged by AD. At present memantine is not available free of charge on the National Health Service.

Prior to the introduction of these drugs the outlook for people with dementia and those close to them was bleak. At the point of diagnosis the only prospect offered was one of protracted mental decline, potential behavioural problems, including incontinence and aggression, and the unavoidable eventuality of 24-hour nursing care. The only drug treatments available were prescribed to combat undesirable behaviour such as wandering, aggression and agitation, and were borrowed from areas of psychiatry most concerned with younger adults with florid psychosis – the major tranquillisers such as haloperidol, promazine and thioridazine. They offered not hope but some relief for the carer and sufferer largely at the expense of a degree of cognitive function in that their sedative effect, while alleviating undesirable behaviour, suppressed desirable behaviour also.

The existence of drugs for treatment in AD has encouraged carers, nonprofessional carers in particular, to demand more for people with dementia. Since the introduction of the drugs the Alzheimer's Society has led demands for access for everyone and to combat the so-called postcode lottery that meant some but not all sufferers could avail themselves of treatment free of charge. It is not unfair to say that many carers and indeed people diagnosed with dementia have had to fight, and in many cases continue to fight, for the right to try antidementia drugs and to remain on them once they are prescribed. As a group and as individuals carers have shown that they will not cede to the so-called experts, psychiatrists, doctors, nurses or social workers, but increasingly demand and expect more in the way of treatment, more in the way of quality care and more in the way of equal rights for people with dementia. This is certainly a change in the traditional role expected of people with dementia and informal carers.

The arguments as to the effectiveness of antidementia drugs will continue, NICE will review the use and free availability of such drugs and professionals will argue about their effectiveness. However, the advent of these drugs alone is driving and will continue to drive the search for further treatments and cure not only for AD but for all causes of dementia. Debate concerning the drugs has mobilised carers and people with dementia in a way previously not witnessed as they begin to demand their voices be heard in matters that concern them. It is this eventuality that brings hope to the specialism and that contributes to the cycle for improving care and outcomes, driving change to benefit people living with dementia.

CHALLENGES TO THE MEDICAL MODEL

It has already been seen that because of the nature of the behaviour of people with dementia their care was originally consigned to the asylums and thus became the province of medicine and psychiatry. The 1844 report of the Metropolitan Commissioners in Lunacy insisted that the 'professed and indeed the main object of a county asylum is, or ought to be, the cure of insanity'. With little in the way of treatment for most mental illnesses and none for dementia this goal was obviously unachievable, and those suffering with dementia became the hopeless cases. Relegated to the backwater wards of the large psychiatric institutions, people with dementia and those looking after them were considered the Cinderella branch of mental health services. Despite an inability to cure or treat dementia a medical model of care was pursued and by the 1980s was very much the established model under which care for people with dementia was delivered.

Lacking realistic cure or treatment, the medical model as applied to care of those with dementia was based in a custody and care philosophy. Professionals, doctors (primarily psychiatrists) and nurses (primarily registered mental nurses), were the experts and family and other carers were encouraged to accept the eventuality of custodial care and the handing over of care to the specialists sooner rather than later. Carers who showed determination to keep the person with dementia at home throughout the duration of their disease were viewed as foolhardy, naïve and from the professionals' perspective 'difficult'. For those who persevered in providing home care little in the way of practical assistance was available from either health or social services. The burden of attempting to care in the home in these unsupported circumstances frequently led many carers back to the psychiatrists and nurses, thus perpetuating the assumption of medical expertise in dementia care.

In hospitals and private care homes wards were large and staff few. The focus of nursing care was on meeting needs for nutrition and cleanliness in the quickest time possible. It was considered important that patients were quiet and calm. Disruptive behaviour was by and large treated pharmaceutically, with drugs borrowed from adult psychiatry, the so-called major tranquillisers: chlorpromazine, promazine, thioridazine and haloperidol among them.

The primary shortcoming of the medical model is that it focuses attention on the disease process and little or no attention is given to the individual's experience. In many chronic illnesses, for example cancer, the approach has become more than medical as individuals with the disease have interjected their own experience and demanded their experience be considered. Their cooperation and agreement in the caring relationship was incorporated into care practices at their insistence. For people with dementia this has been slow to happen, largely because it was long held that people with dementia had no experience. People with dementia no longer knew who they were or what was happening to and around them, they had no concept of self it was presumed and even if they did they could not be involved in useful dialogue about it.

For many of us working with people with dementia discourse on the concept of self would not be a subject considered pertinent to our work. Neither, should we decide to investigate, would we find such discourse easily accessible. However, rudimentary understanding of theory in relation to a sense of self and the retention of a sense of self in people who have dementia is key to understanding the importance of new research and thinking about how we approach care of people with dementia and why such abstract theories are driving change in care practice.

In the second edition of his text *Understanding Dementia* (1992) Jacques observed: 'At the final stages the patient may be assumed to have no real subjective awareness, no sense of self at all, and to be in this sense mentally dead.' Jacques continues that 'We could conclude that it does not therefore matter what we do to a severe dementia sufferer, for she will not understand or react. This is tempting, but it is not humane.' While Jacques goes on to urge his readers to adopt the humane approach, in reality pressure of time, lack of resources and the overwhelming demand of tasks to be achieved frequently means that the temptation to administer care to suit the carer and the care environment rather than the cared for is overwhelming.

The assumption that a person who has lived with dementia for a long time and who is considered to be severely cognitively impaired has no sense of self is the premise that has allowed the perpetuation of the medical model and allowed the temptation to behave in ways that are not humane to be perpetuated in care practice. People with dementia, when not perceived as sentient, feeling persons, are treated as objects to be kept clean, fed and quiet. How this is achieved matters little as the object of this care does not experience life as you or I would. This excuses medical personnel from having to address issues other than the disease process. This does not mean that carers can be unkind, simply that interpersonal relationships and care that is negotiated between carer and cared for is not considered necessary. We must, however, also acknowledge that caring in such a manner affords the subject of care no say in what happens to them and denies them the right to be treated as fully fledged human beings. Such an environment is ripe for fostering behaviour that is abusive. The damage of the medical approach is that it narrows our vision of what dementia means to the individual down to dementia alone, discounting the necessity for individual care. The conclusion therefore is that all people with dementia are the same, they need the same things and it does not matter what we do to achieve meeting their needs because they do not know what is happening to them anyway.

By the late 1980s challenges to the medical model on two fronts began to garner attention. Both bore the influence of Professor Tom Kitwood, a psychologist working in Bradford, England. While his name has become synonymous with person centred care approaches he was not alone at this time in calling for, firstly, recognition that a sense of self persists despite dementia and, secondly, that any individual's presentation with dementia cannot be accounted for by dementia alone.

The argument that Kitwood (1997) and his peers pose is that people with dementia, despite progressive cognitive loss, *do* retain a sense of self and *do* feel both emotionally and physically what is happening to them. When we understand and fully accept this it will begin to matter very much how we negotiate care with people who have dementia and how we achieve and prioritise our care practice. It will make changes in our behaviour and how we develop and deliver care approaches inevitable. At the core of these arguments is the premise that the individual's experience is as important as, if not more important than, the process of the disease and that the individual cannot be reduced to being viewed in terms of disease only. Kitwood (1997) asserted that the pathology of dementia alone cannot account for individual presentation with dementia. As Stokes (2000) identifies in respect of people with dementia, 'If the signs and symptoms of dementia are the direct result of the brain pathology, why are they not all compliant and quiet, or all noisy and aggressive?'

Kitwood proposed that a wider explanation of dementia was necessary, one that took other aspects of the individual into account, which sought not just a biological explanation for what was happening to the person. Kitwood also illustrated through his description of the negative interactions between carers and people with dementia the damage that the continuing application of the medical model is causing to individuals with dementia. A more thorough review of Kitwood's work and person centred care is discussed in Chapter 3.

There can be little doubt that the challenge issued by Kitwood to the medical model has been at the forefront of the drive for change in care practice and service development for people with dementia. Over 10 years later we are just beginning to understand the enormity of the change required and the strength of the barriers to achieving that change. However, one thing is clear: this demand for change from a medical approach will not reduce over time and the growth in research evidence will become louder in insisting that it must occur. Kitwood (1997) was insightful when he referred to this change as a change in the culture of care, for change in culture is notably difficult to accomplish.

Bottom-up drivers for change come from within the care specialism, from practitioners realising that what they are doing is not necessarily what they should be doing. By investigating alternative ways, questioning their actions and measuring their efforts against the outcomes of those efforts, they will try to judge whether their efforts are appropriate and use their questioning to decide whether the outcomes are appropriate. This questioning raises several concerns: will our actions produce the desired outcomes and are the outcomes we are striving for appropriate to the expressed needs of those our actions impact upon? In dementia care these questions are increasingly being informed by consultation with people who have dementia and this is very new and very challenging, particularly because it is becoming quite clear through this consultation that we have been acting in ways that have not produced positive outcomes for people who have dementia. The demand this creates for change is huge and surely cannot be ignored; we must acknowledge the need for change and find ways to overcome the barriers to achieving that change. At the same time we have to continue the questioning, continue the consultation and pursue further change. The process of improvement is dynamic in the sense that it is not finite; there is no end but a cycle of continuous change. This is new and in many respects threatening to those of us who have been working in dementia care for more than a few years because it demands skills we have not previously used and highlights the shortcomings of our, not insignificant, efforts thus far.

Evidence for Practice

Bottom-Up Drivers for Change in Dementia Care

Openness concerning diagnosis and the personal impact of dementia by well-known public figures has led to a reduction in stigma, increase in others seeking diagnosis and the empowerment of persons with dementia, together with raising public awareness and funds for research

The activity of the Alzheimer's Society has influenced the way dementia is viewed, contributed to the inclusion of the voice of people with dementia and their carers and ensured those charged with designing and funding services hear that voice

The growth of a research base is leading to the experiences of people with dementia informing practice

Developments in the pharmaceutical industry have not only brought the advent of real treatment but have introduced hope that drives investigation and change

Challenges to the medical model, demanding acknowledgement of all the factors impacting on an individual's experience of dementia, require major and most urgent change

---

TOP-DOWN DRIVERS FOR CHANGE

GOVERNMENT POLICY

Government strategy in the form of Department of Health policy has wrought, arguably, as important a change as the drive for person centred care. A multiplicity of change in a comparatively short space of time includes community care, diploma education for nurses, clinical governance, evidence-based practice, National Service Frameworks and Standards of Care, to name but a few. These directives have taken the care profession and dementia care as an element of that in many new directions, each demanding change in those undertaking to develop and deliver care.

As early as 1961 the then health minister Enoch Powell (1961) called for the closure of the asylums and a move to care in the community. Government papers and legislation from this time on, no matter which political party held sway, culminating in the NHS and Community Care Act (1990) set out to shut down the large psychiatric hospitals and develop services based within local communities. Local authorities, in partnership with health service and independent sector agencies, became responsible for assessing need, designing care packages and ensuring delivery of care for people with mental health needs.

The arguments for and against care in the community continue. Those supporting community care hold that asylum treatment is inhumane, it promotes dependence and institutionalisation and further that by isolating people with mental illness from the community social integration is hampered, stigma increased and disturbed behaviour more likely to persist. Those in favour of retaining the institution or elements thereof cite money saving as the true source of such movement and charge that society is neither ready for nor content to have the mentally ill living among them.

In attempting to draw a baseline of British public opinion prior to the Royal College of Psychiatrists antistigma campaign, Crisp et al. (2000) gave some credence to this view. They found that people with mental health problems continue to be endowed with negative characteristics including being a danger to others, being unpredictable and difficult to talk to. With such views held commonly it is hard to see how people with mental health problems can be accepted, let alone supported and cared for, by the local community. It could be construed that the original reasons for society isolating mentally ill people in out-of-town asylums, that is for the protection of the majority, still persist in the eyes of a large section of society and that rather than isolating people with a psychiatric diagnosis in a large out of town hospital we are now merely isolating them within society. Has a move to community care meant care by the community or care by professionals in the community?

For those trying to offer care to people with dementia political motive and argument is of little importance. The outcome of this political manoeuvring, however, is. The primary objective of community care is to keep people with mental health problems, dementia included, at home for as long as possible. Social and health community services are available to enable that to happen. Whether they are there in adequate numbers and with appropriate resources is open to debate.

The closure of the asylums has had implications for both carers and the cared for. Professionals in dementia care are much less likely to be ward or hospital based. Professionals now work in the community where new skills in assessing and providing for needs within the home environment are demanded or they staff the many private nursing and residential homes that currently provide for the continued need of people with dementia for 24-hour care.

More recent National Health Service (NHS) policy (Department of Health 1997, 1998) has aimed to improve the quality of care through a system of clinical governance and specific frameworks for meeting the needs of a defined service or care group. For people with dementia the National Service Framework for Older People (2001) is the means through which standards are established to drive up quality and ensure equity of service in dementia care. It is not an exact fit, particularly for those under the age of 65 who have dementia, but given that the framework standards require the meeting of specific milestones and that progress is audited there is hope that positive change in care practices will result. Much of this policy also requires service user involvement, necessitating consultation with people with dementia about existing services, while developing new services and working towards empowering people with dementia within the service. This would certainly change the focus of the way in which care is traditionally delivered.

While in theory the claims of government policy in benefiting people with mental health can be well supported, questions can be raised concerning whether or not these benefits have been or can be realised. Top down drivers for change have the power to have a pervasive influence on the quality of the life of people living with dementia and those close to them. It is vital in pursuing the care in the community policy that strategies are put in place to ensure services are developed consistent with need and that services are equitable and accessible throughout the country and realistically resourced both financially and from a human resource point of view. There needs also to be consideration of the impact upon professional carers that these directives entail. Nurses, as the traditional care providers, are now required to work in the community and to concentrate on different aspects of patient need. They are required also to work in partnership with other service providers and family carers; they must cede some of the power they have previously been endowed with as the recognised experts of care. It cannot be presumed that all nurses are happy with the change in direction that this necessitates or that the skills they have are easily transferable. However, again it must be acknowledged that the demands made by NHS directives are driving and will continue to drive a significant need for change in dementia care services.

THE NURSING PROFESSION

Changes within nursing's controlling body have altered approaches to care. As early as 1972 the Briggs report encouraged a research base for the nursing profession, from training through to practice and management. By the 1980s criticism of nurse training and practice together with serious concerns about difficulties in recruitment led to new proposals to overhaul nurse training and steps were taken towards incorporating a research base into that training. The so-called Project 2000 took nurse education from the local hospitals where practice and theory were delivered together to the university and diploma education. Student nurses gained true student status and it was hoped by the then governing body, the United Kingdom Central Council for Nursing, Midwifery and Health Visiting (1986), that they would be taught to 'demonstrate an appreciation of research and use relevant literature and research to aid practice'. They became supernumerary to the staffing complement, and were there to observe and learn. Other changes in nursing led by both government and the governing body, The Nursing and Midwifery Council (NMC), have sought to consolidate this academic, professional approach. The NMC Code of Practice demands that nurses keep their knowledge and skills up-to-date throughout their working lives and conditions of re-registration include evidence of this through the post-registration and practice (PREP) standards and guidelines (Nursing and Midwifery Council 2004). The expectation is one of a nursing workforce that is dynamic and progressive. While this training has been criticised for producing newly qualified nurses who are lacking in practical experience and skills, it also produces nurses who no longer consider themselves handmaiden to the medical staff and who are able to question the status quo.

This should be good news for dementia care where the application of the medical model has for so long had detrimental effects on an individual's care experience and the stagnation of care practices. It should ensure that newly qualified nurses have an awareness of up-to-date research and have basic skills required to incorporate this research into their practice. Given the growing wealth of research concerning care of people with dementia, a pattern of positive change should be well established in care settings.

The difficulty with this process is that by bringing nurse education to university standard many prospective nurses will ask whether the effort would not be better spent gaining a qualification that leads to higher paid employment where the hours are more sociable, the work less responsible and where a true career path can be forged. The trouble with nurse career paths currently being offered is that the higher you go the less contact there is with the patient.

Conferring student status upon nursing students has also led to widespread criticism. Prior to Project 2000 nurses in training comprised a significant element of the NHS workforce. They were expected to complete chores as effectively as nursing assistants and develop clinical and management skills as they progressed. For doing so they were paid a wage roughly equivalent to that of the nursing assistant. While this training was built on tradition rather than a research base student nurses soon discovered whether undertaking basic care requirements such as taking people to the toilet, bathing and dressing was how they wished to spend their working lives. Project 2000 students were afforded less opportunity to do so and usually avoided much direct care until qualification, by which point they often perceived their role as telling others how to do it rather than doing it themselves. More and more direct hands-on care became the preserve of the least qualified and poorest paid care team members, the health care assistant. Such a situation, it could be argued, leads to these team members receiving too much in the way of direction and not enough role modelling and direct supervision.

Amendments to Project 2000 have acknowledged this and attempted to redress the balance, but many of the difficulties presently facing the health care industry can be explained as a result of training nurses to challenge tradition and understand research but not giving them sufficient skills to translate this to practice or to instil in many a desire to undertake the basic requirements of nursing care. Indeed, in part this may account for the growing level of a research and anecdotal evidence base in dementia care while care practices overall seem not to be changing at all.

On a more positive note there is widespread agreement that increasingly nurses now have the ability to interpret research and that the volume of research on nursing practice is growing. What appears to be lacking is a method of change management that transforms this *knowing* into *doing*. It is certainly not enough for nurses to know the best method of undertaking clinical practice; they must be able to apply the principles in their everyday activity. This issue will be more closely examined in Chapter 10.

The changes that the governing body of the nursing profession have introduced over the past 10 years have impacted on the lives of nurses and the way in which they undertake their work. Any change is open to criticism and changes to nursing are no exception, but closer examination reveals that it is in trying to implement change that difficulties have occurred rather than the substance of that change. We do need nurses to work in new ways, we do need nurses who understand and can apply evidence to practice and who will question their practice and we undoubtedly do need nurses who are educated not only to do the job but to continue to do the job throughout their nursing career.

Nursing is not the only profession that has undergone a transformation in working patterns and professional boundaries. Social workers, occupational therapists and other professionals working in or with health and social services have found accustomed practices increasingly challenged by top-down drivers for change in dementia care.

Evidence for Practice

Top-Down Drivers for Change in Dementia Care

Government policy has shifted care from the large asylums to the community, aiming to keep people with dementia in their own homes for as long as possible

Government directives demand that professionals develop new skills, work in different environments, in partnership with other service providers and in consultation with people who have dementia

NHS standards strive for equity of care underpinned by clinical governance

Throughout policy the involvement of service users is stipulated as a necessity

The NMC requires that nurses are able to interpret and apply research to practice

---

CONCLUSION

The impetus for change in the dementia care specialism comes from many sources, from above in the form of government policy and the directives of professional ruling bodies and from below from those charged with delivering care and those in receipt of care. Demand for change from all these disparate sources will impact on all areas of care: the environment both physical and social, the way in which we perceive and respond to people with dementia and the manner in which we treat individuals and engage them not only in day-to-day care but in planning for their future as individuals and also as service users in order that their comments on what works and what does not work can be used to build ever-improving services. The frustrations for many working with people with dementia is that given the number and import of the drivers for change actual change is very slow in happening. There are pockets of excellent practice which we rightly celebrate and hold aloft to demonstrate the powerful impact that both research and translating research to practice can bring. However, for those of us working in the field and those with dementia experiencing routine care little true positive change has yet taken place.

In many ways the stage is set and the drivers for change are in place and demanding to be acted upon. Some action has been taken: people with dementia are more likely to be consulted in research than was the case 10 years ago, awareness of dementia has increased among the general public, drugs are being offered and more are in development to treat Alzheimer's disease, more money than ever is being spent on research and the stigma associated with old age and dementia is being challenged. The power to manage the level of change yet to be realised, to pull the disparate strands of what we are learning together to ensure that the life and care of individuals with dementia improves, lies within organisations providing services, their directors and their managers. However, on a much more important level that power to positively change the care experience of persons who have dementia lies with each person who chooses to work with people who have dementia.

3 A New Model of Care

INTRODUCTION

This chapter considers the advent of the person centred philosophy of dementia care and the influence that the introduction of a tangible challenge to the medical model for care of people with dementia that this philosophy presents. The chapter begins by briefly considering why the theory we hold with regard to the way we pursue our caring is important, goes on to consider how the medicalisation of dementia care developed and identifies the consequences of pursuing the medical approach for people with dementia. A large part of the chapter is concerned with a summary of some of the main themes of the person centred care philosophy described by Professor Tom Kitwood, concentrating principally on his seminal work (1997) *Dementia Reconsidered*. This summary is an introduction to the main ideas Professor Kitwood put forward in relation to dementia care and persons with dementia, which will hopefully give readers something to take into their current practice and instil a wish to find out more.

THE IMPORTANCE OF THEORY

The word 'theory' can be defined as hypothesis, premise, supposition or assumption. It refers to a collection of thoughts we have on a subject. Since our thoughts govern our behaviour the thoughts and beliefs we hold on certain subjects are significant as they will heavily influence our behaviour in certain situations. Thus the theory we hold when approaching caring practice is central to the outcome of our practice, as the thoughts we have on the subject receiving care will impact on the nature of the care that subject receives. Florence Nightingale is considered the first nurse theorist; her theory was that health could be improved by improving the environment. She set about implementing her theory through employing a model that emphasised a clean environment that was warm, well ventilated, quiet and well lit.

In the world of caring many different theories underpin various models of practice, for example approaches to helping people overcome anxiety can include psychotherapy, behavioural therapy or pharmacotherapy. Each approach has a theory justifying that particular model of care and is carried out by individuals subscribing to that theory, acquiring the skills the model demands and offering their services to people who need them. The people who need them, being recognised as individuals with their own needs, personality and history, will hopefully find the model and practitioner who can best address their individual needs. People with dementia, until quite recently, have had no such opportunity, primarily because one theory of dementia has governed the model of care provided.

The development of treatments and therapeutic approaches for other types of mental illness led to little in the way of change or development for people with dementia or practitioners in that area. The approach holding sway in the dementia care world was (and arguably largely still is) the medical approach.

Simply put, the medical model is based on the theory of physical cause and effect; something causes disease or illness with the effect that the sufferer experiences or displays symptoms that require investigation, treatment and cure. In applying the medical model it is of paramount importance to uncover the pathology of the disease and identify its nature, origin, cause and progression so that specific treatments can be developed and a cure achieved. Those with experience of working with people who have dementia and some knowledge of the disease will already be somewhat uneasy about the appropriateness of fit of this model as a basis from which to offer care to people with dementia.

One very important point to be made about theory in relation to caring practice is that where the theory does not account for the subject of care adequately the nature of the care will be inappropriate, potentially to the point of abuse. Those with experience of working with people with dementia and some knowledge of the disease will already have a sense that in probably no other care area is this truer than in dementia care. Applying appropriate theory is arguably the most important aspect any practitioner must consider in their approach to practice.

THE MEDICALISATION OF DEMENTIA

The identification and initial description of Alzheimer's disease in the first decade of the twentieth century led directly to the categorisation of Alzheimer's (and other dementias by association) as a disease and indeed as a mental illness and to an inevitable medicalisation of dementia. From this point the search was on to describe the pathology of the disease, and all the other identified dementias, in order to understand how the disease progressed and how symptoms could be controlled, eliminated and the disease itself cured. In the hunt it turned out the person with the dementia, the individual as distinct from the signs and symptoms they displayed, was the last to be considered or consulted.

Jacques remarked as recently as 1988 that, 'there are some good reasons for thinking of dementia as an illness', as doing so 'has stimulated research and encouraged attempts at treatment. It has helped make dementia respectable'. While there may be some truth in this, as we considered in the previous chapter, until recently there was little real advance in the search for a cure and treatment for dementia.

What is true is that there have been some very adverse consequences of thinking of dementia as an illness, the main one being that the medicalisation of dementia has resulted in the medicalisation of the individual with it and a narrowing of the focus of approach to both the disease and the individual, where uncovering pathology, seeking the cause, treating symptoms and striving for a cure are the only goals. Everything that the individual with the disease may say or do is explained in terms of their having the disease and therefore requiring no response other than symptom control. In effect, from the point of diagnosis the person with the disease becomes a fully fledged victim of it, having no ability to control or influence the course or outcome of their dementia and dependent on others to control their lives for them. The medical interpretation of dementia is that everything that happens to the patient, the losses, changes in behaviour and emotional expression, is caused by the damage to the brain that dementia brings. It is considered doubtful that the individual has an experience of their condition and circumstances, and even if they have it will be fragmented and soon forgotten. Jacques (1988) illustrates this commonly held belief clearly when he states:

> The patient herself, on the other hand, is unlikely to be aware of or feel any of these changes in a coherent fashion. She will not recall all the things she used to be able to do and so she will be unable to recognize the change in herself. She will not be able to feel the humiliation of her dependent position.

As we shall see in Chapter 5, research over the past 20 years consistently and clearly refutes this account of the subjective experience of dementia. However, adherence to the medical explanation of dementia has not only delayed investigation of the subjective experience of dementia but prevents current knowledge offered by research from infiltrating practice on a wide enough scale.

Of course, most commentators, including Jacques, urged health professionals not to use the patients' inability to experience what happens to them as an excuse to disregard their need for dignity or to treat them inhumanely. Unfortunately, of course, it is all too easy to ignore this latter piece of advice, particularly under pressure of time. To illustrate, if we believe that people with dementia do not understand, remember or feel what we do to them, then if we are rough, disrespectful and dismissive in our interactions with them does it really matter? This is key when you consider that it is quicker to accomplish care tasks such as washing, dressing and feeding if you do not have to talk to the person you are washing, dressing or feeding and if that person does not complain if you do not wash, dress and feed them in a manner they might find reassuring or similar to the standard they may have been used to before developing dementia. Approaching dementia and people with dementia purely from this perspective places both the dementia care specialism and those with dementia in a hopeless situation. There is no cure and while there may be control of symptoms through use of medication there has long been no treatment for the condition. Furthermore, the medical approach demands a hierarchical structure to care, with the experts, the psychiatric consultants, at the apex and cascading downward through junior doctors, psychiatric nurses and allied health professionals. Family and other carers may have something to add to the structure of care but must defer to the experts, people with dementia themselves have nothing to contribute by virtue of their having dementia. The person with dementia is consequently consigned to the waiting room of medical science, in anticipation of the discovery, at some point in the future, of real treatment or cure for their disease.

The manner in which professional carers are viewed within the mental health specialism under the medical model similarly generates images of hopelessness, where those providing care are largely seen as incapable of working in the more demanding areas of mental health care with people suffering from schizophrenia, bipolar disorder, depression or anxiety. Education, other than in basic physical care and pharmaceutical control of undesirable behaviour, has traditionally been denied to these practitioners on the basis that it was not required. Those considered dynamic and ambitious were rarely found in the milieu of dementia care.

It could almost be understandable that doctors and psychiatrists allied themselves closely to the medical approach to dementia care, for it is ingrained in their training. As Double (2001) identifies: 'Medical students are not primed to realise that human behaviour may not follow rules of physical cause and effect. By the time trainees start psychiatric training they have been firmly indoctrinated in the belief that people can be explained and predicted.' What is more difficult to understand is that other professionals, particularly nurses, accepted without question for so long that the medical model provided an appropriate premise and theory to address the needs of individuals with dementia, specifically because the level and nature of the contact between nurses and the people in their care gave them evidence from their own experience that the model was not appropriate. However, it seems what the profession as a whole elected to do was to buy into the medical approach by assuming that what they witnessed in the behaviour of people with dementia, rather than being reflective of the experience that person was having, was demonstrative of the effect of the dementing disease. The intermittent expression of rational comment, of appropriate emotion or behaviour deemed impossible for their cognitive state were designated erroneous or flashes of insight that could not be sustained.

We can track the resolute adherence by nurses to the model through textbooks and journal discourse on dementia from the 1900s onwards. Most texts on dementia and nursing people with dementia, particularly pre-1990s, illustrate this narrowing of focus and the dismissal of the need to engage with or consider the experience of the individual. In 1957 Altschul and Simpson suggested that the help a nurse could offer should be concerned in the main with the preservation of the patients' social appearance, as this would also help the family of the patient to cope, they advised. Trick and Obcarskas (1968), whose text was used to tutor student nurses, advised that the treatment of dementia was 'Primarily directed at curing the underlying condition. But in addition it is often necessary to try and control the mental symptoms.'

As the mental symptoms were restlessness, agitation and apprehension, they were best controlled through use of major tranquillisers, they advised. Nursing was seen largely as an activity that responded to and managed problems created by the patients' symptoms. Trick and Obcarskas devote a section of their book to 'the special nursing problems of the restless and confused'. They compare the confused patient to a small child waking in a dimly lit room, fearful of bogey men and hobgoblins, the role of the nurse being to provide 'some anchor of stability to which they can cling'. Of course the more severe cases, they cautioned, will require sedation.

In 1988 Jacques stated, with some confidence, that 'the whole problem-orientated approach can transform the attitudes of those working with dementing people from a pessimistic despair to an optimistic but realistic commitment'. The labour of caring for people with dementia was divided into the nursing role of managing behaviour and solving problems, while the more difficult situations were referred to the expert, namely the psychiatrist, for consideration, which generally resulted in prescriptions for tranquillisers.

The care and containment offered to the mentally ill by the workhouses and early asylums was a not too distant relative. Perhaps the best piece of educative advice offered to the nurses of the 1970s came from Trick and Obcarskas, who informed the nurses of the 1970s that the relationship of the nurse to her patient could best be summarised in the phrase 'do unto others as you would be done by'. It is a sad reflection of the development of a dementia care specialism that many clinicians continue to pound this maxim as the basis of their practice. The truth is that given the research developments of the past 20 years and the advances in our understanding of dementia and its experience this maxim is woefully inadequate in describing what it is we need to be able to do in our practice and in our relationship with people who have dementia.

Evidence for Practice

A Medical Approach to Dementia Care

The aim of the medical approach is to define the pathology of the disease, uncover its origin, describe its progression, treat the symptoms and find a cure

There is no cure for dementia and therefore no hope for people with it

No explanation for anything the person says or does is required beyond the fact that they have dementia

Nursing care is concerned with problems – observing them and managing them

Management of behaviour that causes nurses problems is primarily through use of tranquillising medication

The person with dementia has no awareness of what is happening to or around them; therefore it matters little how they are treated, other than treating them humanely

Professional care is provided by those not competent enough to work in other areas of mental health care; the need for education other than in physical care is redundant

---

A NEW APPROACH

It would be untrue to state that all researchers and commentators accepted the absolute truth of the medical explanation of dementia; there were those who questioned this narrow account of the cause and effect of dementia, indeed some who argued that dementia was not a psychiatric diagnosis at all. These commentators questioned that neuropathology was the sole factor involved in the dementing process; rather they proposed that an interaction of neurological and other influences, namely psychological and social, provides a more realistic account of dementia. Although such challenges were not taken seriously there had been concern in many quarters that explaining dementia from a medical perspective exclusively left important questions unanswered. The prime question was that if neurological damage caused by dementia was the sole explanation for what happened to people with dementia why, at postmortem, did the extent of damage to the brain not reflect the extent of dementia the individual exhibited prior to death? What was found was that some people who had presented as severely demented might have only minimal neurological damage while someone who had presented with apparently mild dementia, at post mortem might be found to have extensive neuropathology. It was a contradiction that medical science chose largely to ignore.

One commentator took on the challenge; where his predecessors had questioned the standard explanation of dementia he not only set out the problems with the accepted model but offered an alternative. This commentator, Professor Tom Kitwood, laid out a theory of dementia and a model of caring for people with dementia that not only provides a more acceptable account of dementia but offers methods of establishing caring relationships that can generate hope and secure a better quality of life for those living with dementia and those providing for their care. What Professor Kitwood also did was to lay an immense challenge before the care service, because there was little in the care practices that had gone before that would prepare the practitioner for the nature of the caring processes Professor Kitwood identified as requisite to accomplish the task of successfully meeting the needs of individuals who have dementia in the manner his approach demands.

Professor Kitwood came to the world of dementia care relatively late in his career, but vitally brought with him none of the preconceptions or learned presumptions that many new initiates to the world of dementia care either already have or quickly acquire. As his thinking was untarnished by the prevailing attitudes toward dementia and the accepted care practices he was well placed to offer an objective view of the state of dementia care and describe a new philosophy and approach to caring for people with dementia. A psychologist by training and having a career hitherto concentrated on counselling, ethics and psychotherapy, Professor Kitwood offered an explanation of dementia that sought to put the individual first and central to care, to understand the individual's subjective experience and to find out how the individual is sustained, respected and recognised within relationships, particularly the caring relationship. Professor Kitwood identified how negative interactions offered by carers can undermine an individual's sense of being and self, and offered an account of dementia that included not only neuropathology but social and psychological factors. By his own admission his theories were initially considered tantamount to heresy, but they are both the foundation and cornerstone of what we know as person centred care (PCC). Professor Kitwood's theories on dementia, what it means to be a person, the malignant effects of some care practices on the person with dementia and the nature of the caring relationship, are described below.

DEMENTIA

We have seen that the medical model of care identifies dementia as a disease process causing neurological change that leads to the set of signs and symptoms we term 'dementia'. The requirement is for medical science to investigate the cause, seek treatment and develop a cure; while such developments are awaited the role of carers is to provide the physical care increasing dependence requires and to cope with problematic behaviour that is part of the disease process. As other commentators suggested, explaining dementia in this way discounts the influence of the many factors that impact on an individual. These influences do not suddenly cease when a person develops dementia, but have an effect on the way in which the individual copes with and expresses themselves when they have dementia. Professor Kitwood used an equation to summarise these influences:

$$D = P + B + H + NI + SP$$

In the person centred model of dementia care D or dementia is seen as the sum of the individual's Personality, Biography or life story, their physical Health, Neurological Impairment and Social Psychology, the social and physical context within which the individual lives. It is these factors that determine the pattern of a person's experience of dementia and how this is expressed. If we consider again the medical model we see that NI and H are the only factors given consideration in caring for the person. However, Professor Kitwood's account acknowledges that the individual's personality, all that has gone before in their life, the things that they have done and achieved, their environment, relationships, standards of living their life and the way in which they spend time are of the utmost importance in understanding how a particular individual presents with dementia.

This then is the first step in PCC – understanding the influences on the individual in order that we can better understand the person and meet their needs within the caring relationship. Getting to know the individual and their biography, often to the point of helping them to reconstruct their life story, is one of the key elements to PCC. Similarly, assessing the impact of the person's social and physical environment and the way in which it impacts on the individual is paramount.

THE PERSON IN PCC

The concept of what it means to be a person and how a person should be treated, related to and communicated with is central to PCC. Professor Kitwood subtitled his influential work (1997) 'The Person Comes First'. In part this was to emphasise the manner in which the needs of the individual are marginalised under the medical model and in part to indicate a way of understanding just what can be achieved if *person* replaces *disease* as the focus of care approaches.

That each person has absolute value and that each individual is unique, sensitive and worthy of respect is a common philosophical theme that we all generally recognise and accept, but we might not understand the processes that enable a person to feel that they are valuable, unique or individual. In order to understand this we have to consider the importance of relationships. Professor Kitwood suggests that in human life there is an interdependence and interconnectedness between individuals. In terms of social psychology, the place of the individual in society and the roles they hold, their sense of self and how this is maintained and integrated is bound up with this interdependence and connectedness, which in turn is played out in the relationships we have with others. The importance of relationship then is that our experience within relationships can confirm or deny that we are unique, sensitive, valuable human beings deserving of respect. Professor Kitwood describes this concept as 'personhood' and defines it as 'a standing or status that is bestowed upon one human being, by others, in the context of relationship and social being. It implies recognition, respect and trust'.

If an individual or a specific group of individuals are not accorded personhood and are not respected as unique individuals, if they are considered less unique, individual or deserving of the respect of others, in effect the individual or group of individuals becomes dehumanised. Professor Kitwood suggests this happens to groups in society who are severely disabled, including the aged and those with dementia. He points out also that the consequences for individuals and groups of individuals can be detrimental. For people with dementia specifically, the lack of adequate services, in terms of resources or appropriate training in the interpersonal skills required to ensure good psychological care, is a result. Furthermore, this dehumanisation together with the particular anxieties others feel in relation to dementia, namely the fear of frailty and dependence and the fear of going mad, have led to what Professor Kitwood describes as a 'malignant social psychology', a relegation of people with dementia to the realms of unbeing, where their sense of self is lost and the need to treat them as others are treated is unnecessary.

If we reflect on how our theory of something affects the way we behave, we can now see that if we believe that people with dementia do not need to be regarded as individuals who are unique, valuable and human then the way in which we treat them will be very different from the way in which we relate to people whom we acknowledge as full human beings. It is important to remember that it is not just poor practitioners who respond to people with dementia as if they are less human than others. Potentially good practitioners who subscribe to a theory of dementia that places the disease and the disease process at the centre of care will struggle to reconcile what they know about dementia with a requirement to apply specialist skills in developing relationships that support and sustain an individual's personhood.

The person centred philosophy acknowledges that despite a loss of memory, loss of reasoning skills, loss of ability to communicate clearly and loss of capacity to make and take action on decisions the individual with dementia remains a human being. The challenge for carers is to incorporate this belief into their practice and to behave in relationships with people who have dementia in a manner that reflects this belief and strives to uphold their personhood. As Professor Kitwood states in good care 'identity remains intact because others hold it in place'. Thus good care is that which enables the person with dementia to know who they are, that they are valuable and unique and that they know this because the way in which those around them behave and relate to them confirms this.

MALIGNANT SOCIAL PSYCHOLOGY

If we recognise that the process of good care involves developing and sustaining relationships that demonstrate respect for the individual and reflects our acknowledgement of them as valuable and worthy members of the human race with the aim of upholding and reinforcing that individual's identity, then we must also consider what should happen if we were to fail to do so. Professor Kitwood (1997) reflects on the findings of Meacher in 1972 who concluded that the social psychology of residential homes was enough to 'drive people demented'. In effect, the conclusion is that the psychosocial environment that has been created to care for people with dementia by the process of dehumanising the individual and relating to the individual in a way that detracts from their personhood has the consequence of exacerbating the dementing process. Put in the plainest terms, the traditional approach to dementia care makes dementia worse.

It is this that more realistically accounts for the variance at post-mortem and explains why some people with minimal neurological damage presented as severely demented and some with extensive damage presented as only mildly impaired. Suddenly it becomes very important to consider the way we relate to people with dementia, because if we concur with this line of thought then we understand that we hold a key role in the life of someone living with dementia, the difference perhaps between living successfully with dementia or developing dementia at an increased rate.

Professor Kitwood exemplified the malignant social psychology in dementia care with a list of 17 types of interaction commonly used by those providing care which result in the depersonalisation of the person with dementia and the potential exacerbation of dementia. These interactions serve to disempower, deceive, patronise, intimidate, stigmatise, pressurise, invalidate, objectify, mock, disturb and reduce the individual to less than human.

The sobering aspect for all of us who have worked in dementia care for any length of time is that we can recognise ourselves in the behaviour described by Professor Kitwood. It is not just intentionally abusive people who abuse people who have dementia; unintentional abuse in the context of relationships exists. I know because I have behaved in this way. Of course, once the consequences of the behaviour become clear and are understood there is no excuse for the behaviour to continue, for to continue to contribute to a malignant social psychology once one is aware of the outcome for people who have dementia is to perpetrate abuse intentionally.

THE NATURE OF THE CARING RELATIONSHIP

That an individual with dementia has any subjective experience of life at all is a relatively new concept. The medical model required that no attention be given to what the individual's experience of dementia might be and what was implicitly accepted was an approach based on the old adage that where there is no sense there is no feeling. However, in the late 1980s challenges to this long accepted dictum began to be taken more seriously. Professor Kitwood identified that although there are common elements to the experience of dementia an individual's experience will be coloured by their own personality and life history. Thus some people cope very poorly with the onset of dementia; for some the loss of cognitive ability is devastating and grief provoking while others will seem to cope with the onset of dementia quite ably and progress to have a relatively benign experience of the disease. The importance of uncovering an individual's experience of dementia lies in the access it then gives care practitioners to information to make life with dementia not only bearable but enjoyable and in defining what is needed from practitioners to establish and sustain a relationship with the individual that will enhance their quality of life.

Accessing the subjective experience of dementia is difficult given the communication barriers that dementia brings, but Professor Kitwood suggested seven methods of gaining awareness of what it must be like to live with dementia. These are consulting the writings of individuals who have written about their experience of dementia, listening carefully to what people with dementia say in an interview and group setting, similarly attending to individuals in the course of everyday life, learning from the actions and behaviour of people who have dementia, consulting with others who have experienced illnesses that cause similar symptoms to dementia (meningitis and depression for example), using your own imagination and adopting role play. In this manner we may be able to develop an understanding of what it must be like to live each day with this syndrome, which impacts in such a global way on an individual's life.

Where a medical model of care prevails and a malignant social psychology surrounds individuals with dementia, Professor Kitwood suggests the experience will be only negative, bound up in feelings of fear. Fear of abandonment, of humiliation, of being controlled and imprisoned, where panic and grief are such constant companions that global states of terror, misery, rage and chaos only are possible, leading to permanent states of despair, depression, exhaustion, apathy and a vegetative state. This very negative picture of what it might be like to have dementia stems directly from what we can extrapolate the consequences of not supporting personhood are likely to be. There appears little in the line of research or anecdotal evidence, either before or after Kitwood, to counteract such an extrapolation; indeed the contrary is true.

There is, obviously, an alternative positive outcome when personhood is supported and individuals are respected. This is the essence of person centred care and the focus of the caring relationship. This alternative outcome occurs when an individual's psychological needs are attended to. Through the meeting of psychological needs, Professor Kitwood proposes, the experience of dementia can become positive. The five overriding psychological needs identified by Professor Kitwood are the needs for comfort, attachment, inclusion, occupation and identity. These needs are not hierarchical and none is more important than another; the meeting of one need because it is closely connected to the other has a positive effect on the others. When psychological needs are met an individual feels loved. The vulnerability dementia brings and the inability of the person to seek or initiate support in getting these needs attended to means that for the person with dementia the meeting of these needs is compromised. For the caring relationship, anticipating and supporting these needs is paramount because, as Professor Kitwood states, unless these needs are met 'a human being cannot function, even minimally, as a person'.

If the prime task of caring for a person with dementia is to maintain personhood and the way to maintain personhood is to meet psychological needs then how might we meet psychological needs? The key according to Professor Kitwood lies in the nature of our interactions with people who have dementia. This he termed 'positive person work', a way of interacting that recognises the individual, consults and collaborates with the individual, provides contact and enables play, provides reassurance and pleasure, that celebrates life, encourages relaxation, that validates and generates feelings of being safe and that enables, rather than disables, the person.

Not only did Professor Kitwood believe that poor care actually exacerbates dementia he also put forward the theory that good care can improve dementia. Based on his own experience of working with people who have dementia and the then (in 1997) sparse amount of studies suggesting that a level of 'rementia' (reversal of dementia) was possible, he predicted that the accepted theory of dementia, that it is solely a neurodegenerative disease, would be proved false. He suggested that developing good dementia care is 'not just a matter of providing the very best of palliative care, but actually reshaping the course of neurodegenerative disease'. If proved correct he proposed that 'The door would then be open for a radical reconstruction of the whole field, giving dementia care an immensely more important place.'

What is being proposed is that if the traditional approaches to caring for people with dementia are replaced by practices based on taking a person centred approach, one that is based on supporting personhood and meeting psychological needs, then not only will there be a vast improvement in the quality of life and well-being of persons with dementia but it will be possible to reverse some of the progress of the disease in individuals. In the long term many of the very negative endstage symptoms previously thought to be a consequence of the dementia will prove instead to have been consequences of the negative nature of care practices. As a result the clinical presentation of dementia will have to be rewritten.

CONCLUSION

The great loss to the world of dementia care that Professor Kitwood's death brought in 1998 leaves us to question how much further along the way to proving his theory we might have been had he not died so soon after the publication of his major work on dementia. There can also be no doubt that many, many practitioners are striving daily to put into operation a person centred approach in working with people who have dementia. There can also be no doubt that many researchers are working hard to investigate Professor Kitwood's theories. There are those, an increasing number it seems, who are growing despondent at ever achieving the level of change needed across care settings that would be required to discover whether care practices are so important in shaping the future classification of dementia. The education of practitioners in the interactions required to support personhood has largely been undertaken; few care areas are ignorant of the term person centred care, but there is a perception that little of practical value has changed. While there may be some stunning examples in the form of small projects or individual nursing homes of the success of taking a person centred approach the broad view is not encouraging.

I would suggest that those who are despondent should re-visit Professor Kitwood's work and consider again the extent of the task before us. Professor Kitwood himself described the change required as a change of 'culture'. Although he suggested ways that this could be achieved I would suggest that even he underestimated the size of the task. The scope of new research into the psychosocial aspects of dementia and dementia care and the level at which individual studies lead to yet more areas where research is required give an indication of the size of the task before us. This is a cultural change to be chipped away at, where small gains will be made over long periods of time.

An outline of what is needed from practitioners to begin to incorporate more person centred approaches in their care is provided at the end of the chapter. If tangible change still seems a distant prospect we can only continue to question our own practice, question the scope of our influence and be sure that we are doing the best that we can. The nature and level of skills required to introduce, support and sustain person centred care across the spectrum of organisations that offer that care is phenomenal. What we are experiencing now is merely a reflection of just how huge the job is. If each of us accepts this and continues to use our sphere of influence then positive things can result and a more perceptible change will come.

The frustration comes from concern for individuals currently subject to poor care, from empathy with their suffering and from a desire to wake up the conscience of those perpetrating poor care practices to get them to see the error of their ways. Perhaps it stems most of all from fear that we ourselves will develop dementia before the advent of the new culture of dementia care and that we will at some point have to live in an environment where a malignant social psychology prevails.

Evidence for Practice

What Is Needed from Practitioners of Good Dementia Care?

Recognition that dementia is not explained purely in terms of neuropathology

Understanding that the factors that influence an individual's experience of dementia are the individual's personality, biography, health, neurological impairment and social psychology

Understanding the importance of supporting an individual's personhood, recognising and responding to each person as a human being, with unique identity and worthy of respect

Understanding that poor care practices can exacerbate the progression of dementia by contributing to a malignant social psychology and realising that poor care practices are not the province solely of poor practitioners

Recognition of the importance of understanding what it must be like to have dementia, and fostering the ability to place oneself in the individual's situation in order to come close to their experience

Understanding that the meeting of psychological needs enhances personhood, upholds identity and thus constitutes the primary task of care

Developing skills in interacting with persons with dementia that accomplish the meeting of psychological needs

Recognition that to impact on the life of the person with dementia this positive work must be continuous and pervasive

4   Whose Diagnosis Is It?

INTRODUCTION

A combination of factors including increased accuracy of diagnosis, the development
of pharmaceutical treatment and increased pressure to consult with people with dementia as service users has prompted debate on the need to tell people with dementia
that they have dementia. This chapter looks at the process of reaching a diagnosis
of dementia, the arguments for and against disclosing that diagnosis to the person
and how disclosure may be undertaken and supported. Developing a routine in practice that involves telling people they have dementia has huge implications for future
service development, not least in meeting the needs of people in the early stage of
the disease process when services are traditionally not available. The trend in practice increasingly is to disclose the diagnosis to the individual and a growing body
of evidence supports this practice. If this trend continues, however, those providing
services will need to be responsive to the need for support in coping with receiving
the diagnosis and developing strategies to live with dementia.

DIAGNOSING DEMENTIA

The process of diagnosing dementia is a specialist task and, as we have seen in
Chapter 1, not without complications. However, most commentators concur that the
diagnosis can now be achieved with significant accuracy. The assessment of what
might be dementia is generally coordinated by a psychiatrist with a team comprising
the skills of psychiatric nursing, occupational therapy, physiotherapy, psychology, social work and speech therapy. General practitioners have a role to play in undertaking
routine examinations to rule out obvious causes of symptoms, for example infection,
that may be causing acute confusion and ensuring prompt referral to specialist services to facilitate early diagnosis. Early diagnosis will afford the individual access to
more specialist services and enable them and those close to them to start planning for
a future living with dementia. Equally important is achieving an accurate diagnosis
where dementia is not causing presenting symptoms or where an acute episode is
making symptoms of an existing dementia worse. While investigation into the origin
of symptoms suggestive of a dementia syndrome is a specialist task carers and indeed people with symptoms themselves have a right to request such investigation. In
particular, individuals should be encouraged to seek help rather than putting memory
difficulties down to old age.

The Royal College of Psychiatrists (RCP) (2005) has issued guidelines for the diagnostic assessment and investigation of suspected dementia. Elements of that investigation include expert mental state assessment and assessment of the physical state. The RCP also advises that consideration should be given to factors such as depression, social, family and relationship factors. This latter involves compiling a full history of all activities of daily living, behaviour and abilities, nutritional habits, social situation, relationships and sleep patterns, and how suddenly and severely the symptoms occurred. The information needs to be gathered from the individual with symptoms, those who live with them or those having close contact. Documenting a full history of the nature and development of symptoms is the first step in aiding correct diagnosis and in highlighting what may not be dementia.

This history taking should be added to a full physical and mental state examination undertaken by a physician. The Royal College of Psychiatrists advises the following blood investigations: full blood count, ESR, B12 and folate, urea and electrolytes, calcium, liver function test and glucose test, and, where history taking indicates, tests for syphilis, serum lipids and HIV. A chest X-ray and electrocardiogram may also be carried out. The results of such tests when considered with the history that has been given should reveal any reversible metabolic, endocrine, deficiency and infective states, whether they cause symptoms or exacerbate an existing dementia. Where there are unexplained or rapid onset symptoms or when a history of recent head injury is known a computerised tomography (CT) scan should aid diagnosis and exclude space occupying lesions, large strokes, severe atrophy or intracranial haematoma. The consensus is that age should not be a barrier to such investigations. This is important as in the past rationing of resources has led to such diagnostic techniques being restricted on the basis of age, possibly interfering with the process of correct diagnosis. An electroencephalogram may assist differential diagnosis, particularly where the person experiences altered or fluctuating levels of consciousness or seizures. Genetic testing, although not routinely offered, is undertaken in specialist centres and is important where such a link is suspected.

Together with careful history taking and physical screening an assessment of cognition and mental state is required. The standard test for cognition in older adults is the Mini-Mental State Examination (Folstein et al. 1975), but of itself this tool should not be considered sufficient for a diagnosis of dementia syndrome. The process of diagnosis is one of building a full picture of each individual's strengths and needs. A further aspect of mental state requiring consideration, as discussed in Chapter 1, is the existence of a depressive illness. Depression as we know can appear to share similar symptoms to dementia and a diagnosis of dementia does not exclude the possibility of co-morbid depression. To repeat Clarfield's (2003) advice, whatever is found to be treatable should be treated irrespective of whether what is found is causing symptoms of dementia or complicating an identified dementia.

DEALING WITH THE DIAGNOSIS

Without exception the literature available concerning the diagnosis of dementia highlights the need for early diagnosis. Indeed Standard Seven of the *National Service Framework for Older People* (Department of Health 2001a) demands that early diagnosis is given priority. Dementia as we know is a progressive disease and the consensus seems to be that the sooner it is detected the better. This makes sense if we consider how the person with the disease will want to plan for the future and involve those close to them in considering a future living with dementia. However, it makes little sense if, having been able to diagnose a dementing disease, we then withhold this information from the individual. In practice today it is by no means a foregone conclusion that people with dementia are told that they have dementia. In fact dementia remains one of the few diagnoses that are routinely withheld from the person with it. Although there is some evidence of change in practice around diagnosis disclosure, the traditional route to disclosure in this area is, as with many aspects of dementia care, to approach it by proxy. The diagnosis is given to and discussed with the next of kin or significant others and disclosed to the individual at their discretion and indeed often by them rather than by those who have made the diagnosis. Professionals, who are encouraged by national and local policy to promote inclusion and partnership of and with people with mental health problems and who are more than aware of the rights of the individual to confidentiality of information, feel that they can justify exclusion and breach of confidentiality by virtue of the person's diagnosis.

The development of practice in disclosing a diagnosis of dementia to the patient has frequently been compared to the way in which practice in disclosing a diagnosis of cancer to the individual with cancer changed from the 1960s onward. A comparative study by Novack *et al.* (1979) reveals a complete reversal in attitude and practice by physicians in disclosing a diagnosis of cancer to the patient. When questioned in 1961 90 % of doctors did not tell the patient they had cancer, but by 1977, 97% were disclosing to the patient. A similar shift in attitude and practice is currently underway in the field of dementia care. This should be viewed as a positive change but great care needs to be taken to ensure the guidelines that are developed around the process of disclosure are sensitive to individual need.

Evidence for Practice

Diagnosing Dementia

The diagnosis of dementia is a specialist task involving a full multidisciplinary team

An assessment of the physical and mental state is required together with taking a full history

Diagnosis should eliminate any other cause of symptoms

Where treatable symptoms are found they should be treated

Early diagnosis is essential and prioritised within health standards

REASONS FOR NOT DISCLOSING A DIAGNOSIS OF DEMENTIA

The arguments against disclosing a diagnosis of dementia to the person with it are centred on a desire to shelter them from bad news. It seems that it is generally felt that giving the diagnosis would prompt anxiety and distress in the individual and thus is best to be avoided. This, however, may be more about the anxieties of the individual who is breaking the news to the person and about family who are worried about having to cope with the distress they fear the person will express. There is concern also that knowledge of the diagnosis may trigger depression and even suicidal ideation, although there is no evidence to support these fears. Despite the current accuracy with which diagnosis can be achieved, fears of misdiagnosing are also given as a reason for not passing on the diagnosis. It is also argued that there is little to be achieved by telling the person that they have dementia because they will forget anyway. This forgetfulness fuels reluctance in those who anticipate having to deliver this bad news on more than one occasion. Research studies reflect an interesting anomaly in that carers who were in favour of withholding a diagnosis of dementia felt that were it their own diagnosis they would want to know (Holroyd *et al.* 1996). Similarly, a majority of doctors would also wish to know if they were diagnosed with Alzheimer's disease (Johnson *et al.* 2000).

A close examination of the arguments against disclosure shows them to be on shaky ground. It must be acknowledged that anyone given a diagnosis of dementia is likely to be anxious and upset; it is a life altering diagnosis. Even those with a little knowledge gained from the mass media will understand that the prospect of living with dementia is a daunting one. However, this is not a reason for withholding that information; people with cancer are routinely given their diagnosis and the prospect of receiving that diagnosis is equally shocking. What is needed from us as carers and as people likely to be well placed to disclose the diagnosis is that we anticipate a shocked response and so need to make the disclosure in a manner that will cushion the shock and then respond in a supportive way. This will enable the individual to begin a process of accepting the diagnosis and learning to live with dementia.

The fact that a person could develop depression and become suicidal in response to being told they have dementia cannot be ignored. However, developing depression and considering self-harm may be even more likely if the person undergoes a period of intensive assessments at the hands of several specialists only to be told they are all right. They know they are not all right! Denying individuals the right to know what is wrong with them and denying them a frame of reference for all the worrying things that are happening to them, particularly when those around them remain concerned about their performance and behaviour, could also prompt depression or suicidal ideas. If anything, the increased understanding we have about depression and dementia should prompt us to disclose the diagnosis so that we can form plans of care, including risk management, with the individual to militate against depression and to recognise its manifestation early where it is a feature.

Concern about misdiagnosis as an argument against disclosure is an excuse rather than a reason. The accuracy of establishing a diagnosis of dementia is now upwards of 90 % (Kukull *et al.* 1990), making misdiagnosis unlikely.

The nature of dementia is that the memory of those with it is impaired; on this basis it is argued that delivering bad news is best avoided. This argument works on two levels: firstly, the bad news would not be retained and, secondly, the bad news would have to be delivered repeatedly. This perpetuates a cycle of distress as the person learns again and again, as if for the first time, that they have dementia. It is on this basis that people with dementia are denied all kinds of information, for example the death of a spouse, their admission to hospital or a nursing home and their diagnosis. Good news is not treated in the same way. If a person with dementia becomes a grandparent they are told and if a son or daughter has something to celebrate they are told. It seems that if the news is good it does not matter if it is forgotten and we do not mind repeating it, but if it is bad it should be avoided. This indicates more concern about the impact on the deliverer of news than the nature of the news and requires not the vetting of information but the development of expertise in delivering information. We need to acknowledge that what we are seeking to avoid is the distress we fear might accompany the repetition of a diagnosis of dementia and our own limited ability to put ourselves and the person with dementia through that potentially traumatic experience again and again. This particularly applies to ourselves, as we would be likely to remember the previous occasions and would not want to repeatedly put ourselves in that position again. However, consider the alternative. Presumably we are delivering the diagnosis more than once because the person keeps asking what is wrong with them. If we are to be honest why should we not disclose the diagnosis again? How many times is enough? Should there be a set number of times we tell before it is decided to stop? Better still would be some education and support for carers, both professional and familial, on how to keep delivering this and other bad news repeatedly while avoiding too much stress in themselves and developing more skilful approaches in supporting the individual through the disclosure of bad news.

My own experience in disclosing a diagnosis of dementia is that most people do remember that they have been given an explanation for what is happening to them. Some have difficulty remembering the name, particularly Alzheimer's, but it has not been my experience that the process of disclosure is cyclical and unending. On a personal note the most upsetting issue around disclosure is where family members insist the diagnosis is withheld but the person keeps asking what is wrong with them. This is a much more uncomfortable place to be, as abiding by the family's request involves lying to the person with dementia and the implications for your relationship with that person will be that the relationship cannot be based in trust, the most basic requisite of any therapeutic relationship. We must also consider, as professionals, that when we leave disclosure to the discretion of family carers we are often also leaving the act of disclosure to them. However poorly prepared we, as professionals, are to disclose the diagnosis, surely having such an expectation of family carers is unacceptable.

In a systematic review of the literature on diagnosis disclosure Bamford *et al.* (2004) provide further factors that influence the professionals' practice in this area. They identify that professionals make judgements about the individual's level of dementia and the likelihood of the individual being able to understand and process the information in a useful way. People whose dementia has progressed to advanced stages before diagnosis is achieved are therefore very unlikely to be informed. Bamford *et al.* confirm that the desires of family or other carers play a part in professionals' decisions to divulge diagnosis; where those close to the person with dementia are against disclosure the professional is less likely to disclose.

The arguments against disclosing a diagnosis of dementia to individuals with dementia are well documented in the literature and consist mostly of opinions and fears held by carers both professional and informal. These arguments do not hold up well under close examination and are indicative of our own reservations about having to undertake the act of disclosure and deal with the consequences rather than giving consideration to the ethical or legal rights of the individual whose diagnosis it is or to their possible need for or use of the information.

Evidence for Practice

Factors Contributing to a Decision Not to Disclose Diagnosis

Desire to shelter the individual from bad news

Desire to avoid upsetting the person

Concern that knowledge of diagnosis may prompt depression and suicidal intent

Desire to avoid having to cope with the emotional distress of the person receiving the diagnosis

Belief that the person would not remember

The reluctance of carers or significant others

Fear of misdiagnosis

The severity of the person's dementia

ARGUMENTS IN FAVOUR OF DISCLOSING DIAGNOSIS TO PEOPLE WITH DEMENTIA

Arguments in favour of giving the individual a diagnosis of dementia may be divided into four areas of consideration, each of which is discussed below. These are to provide an opportunity for the person to seek help, to provide an opportunity for them to come to terms with and develop coping strategies in living with dementia, to provide an opportunity for the individual to resolve life issues and to plan for the future and lastly the obligations of professionals to provide correct and timely information to those in their care.

Firstly, the opportunity to seek help or treatment can be supported by telling the individual what is wrong with them. With the knowledge of what is causing their difficulties the person can seek information on drug treatments and alternative therapies. They can investigate what services are available in their area to enable them to live as independently as possible with dementia, and where they may gain emotional support and meet people in similar circumstances to themselves. Knowledge of diagnosis also allows the person to consider becoming involved in research, an opportunity that is increasingly being offered to persons with dementia and vital in progressing both treatment and care approaches. It may also allay fears about passing the disease on to family members where this is not a possibility.

One of the first responses to receiving any negative health diagnosis will be 'What can I do about it?' It is no different when one receives a diagnosis of dementia. One of the driving forces against diagnosis disclosure in the past lies in the professionals' inability to respond with anything positive to this inquiry. However, this is changing. The advent of drug treatments for Alzheimer's disease is one avenue of hope, but research and advances in developing interpersonal relationships and theories on coping with dementia now afford the professional more positive outcomes to offer following diagnosis disclosure.

The second consideration, that disclosure will support the individual in coming to terms with dementia, is a relatively new phenomenon. Only 10 to 15 years ago raising a point in favour of disclosing a diagnosis of dementia on the basis that it allowed the person the opportunity to come to terms with it would have been considered ridiculous. The development in our understanding of the subjective experience of dementia, together with a growing body of evidence supporting the ability of the individual to develop and use coping strategies, now makes it a necessity.

People who have dementia know that something is wrong. They may be distressed by what is happening, they may make excuses for their change in behaviour or performance, they may avoid situations that highlight their inability to do what they used to do, they might ignore the difficulties dementia brings or encourage their spouse or relatives to collude with them to cover up and they may blame others close to them for what is happening. People respond in different ways to having dementia, but they do know something is wrong. The response to having dementia is similar to having other life changing diseases and, as with other life changing diseases, knowledge of the diagnosis, an explanation of what it is that is changing their life, will offer the opportunity to come to terms with and to begin to live with the disease. Kitwood (1997) identified the process of grief that accompanies dementia as people mourn the loss of the abilities they had. This occurs whether or not the individual has a name to attach to that loss, but increased awareness of what is happening against a background of helping services aimed at enabling individuals to learn to live with dementia is important and is one of the ways forward for the development of a specialist dementia care service.

Thirdly, we should consider that knowledge of the diagnosis gives the individual the chance to resolve outstanding issues in life and to consider their desires for the future. Whether this is repairing family relationships, making practical plans with regard to finances and accommodation, achieving a once in a lifetime ambition sooner rather than later or making their wishes for end of life care known through advance directives, the importance of offering this chance should not be underestimated. In relation to many future decisions the difficulties of approaching such subjects now will be outweighed by the benefits of knowing what the person wants when the point comes where they are not in a position to easily communicate wishes to family and carers. Having such information at a later stage will be invaluable for the professional care team and save the family having to address very painful issues at very stressful times. It is a way to try and ensure that the individual's wishes are known and adhered to beyond the time when they are deemed to have the capacity to make decisions.

Finally, in support of disclosing the diagnosis is the perspective from the professional position. The universal right of the individual to medical information about themselves and the obligation of professionals in possession of that information to pass it on to the individual are supported in the literature on medical ethics (Hebert *et al.* 1997) and encouraged in Department of Health (DoH) policy through service user involvement initiatives. DoH policy endorses the philosophy of patient involvement, including people with dementia, in documents such as the *National Service Framework for Older People* (Department of Health 2001a) and *Shifting the Balance of Power: The Next Steps* (Department of Health 2002). In this latter document the DoH calls for radical cultural and organisational change that will empower patients to 'become informed and active partners in their care involving them in the design, delivery and development of local services'. This cannot realistically be achieved in a care environment where diagnosis is routinely withheld from the patient.

The Nursing and Midwifery Council Code of Practice (2004), the standards by which nurses undertake their practice, requires that nurses recognise that 'All patients and clients have a right to receive information about their condition' and further that they 'Should seek patients' and clients' wishes regarding the sharing of information with their family and others.' It should not be the other way around, which is traditionally the approach taken in the care of the person with dementia. Hebert *et al.* also point to truth telling with regard to diagnosis as being not only about enabling decision making but as a means to fostering trust in the patient's relationship with the professional and demonstrating the respect owed to the patient as a person.

Those providing services are continually urged to be person centred in their approach, to place the individual receiving care at the centre and in a position of control of that care. To claim adherence to these principles while withholding the truth with regard to diagnosis is a nonsense.

Informing the individual that they have dementia keeps them 'in the loop', within that circle of people who are affected by the disease and in communication with the people who have the skills and tools to do something about it. This knowledge allows the person to grieve for what they are losing, to share this sorrow with family and those close to them and to begin life with dementia in as prepared a way as is possible. That is not to say that the process is easy, but reinforces the fact that disclosing a diagnosis of dementia to the person with dementia is necessary. We are beginning to develop practice in disclosing the diagnosis and there are examples of good and bad practice that we can learn from. Listening to people who have dementia will be invaluable in informing this area of practice, but what little research has thus far been undertaken with people who have dementia indicates their desire to know what is wrong with them.

Evidence for Practice

Arguments in Favour of Disclosing Diagnosis

Provides an opportunity for the individual to consider possible treatment

Offers an opportunity for the individual to consider becoming involved in research

Allows an opportunity for the individual to seek psychosocial support

Provides the individual with an opportunity to resolve life issues and to plan for the future

There is a professional obligation to give information to patients and not to give it to others without the individual's express permission

People with dementia know something is wrong so withholding diagnosis may be harmful

Individuals have a right to information about themselves

SHOULD EVERYONE WITH DEMENTIA BE TOLD THEY HAVE DEMENTIA?

The research conducted with people with dementia on the subject of whether a diagnosis of dementia should be disclosed is sparse. However, what there is reinforces not only the desirability of disclosure but the need for haste of disclosure. Pratt and Wilkinson (2001) found that people with dementia want to know their diagnosis and they want to know as soon as possible in order that they can make best use of their time and the positive opportunities afforded by disclosure. Further studies undertaken with older adults without dementia who were asked whether they would want to know if they developed dementia revealed that an overwhelming majority would wish to know (Erde *et al.* 1988; Holroyd *et al.* 1996).

Calls for early detection of dementia are universal in literature and research about dementia. This is primarily because it is before the disease advances that the individual has the best opportunity to prepare themselves and their family for its effects.

However, what about those individuals for whom the diagnosis is later in coming, whose dementia is quite advanced before diagnosis is sought or established? Professional carers experience an ethical dilemma when they know the person's right to diagnosis but they perceive that telling the truth will harm the patient. In the care of the person with dementia this can be extreme as the perception may be that the individual will have the ability to understand the diagnosis and the implications of having dementia, but not have the ability to develop coping strategies or to come to terms with having such a progressively debilitating syndrome. As Pinner (2000) highlights, there are parallels between diagnosis disclosure in the field of cancer care and dementia care, but with dementia altering the person's cognition, judgement and insight issues around disclosure are different.

Arguments in favour of disclosing a diagnosis to the person with dementia certainly appear to outweigh the disadvantages, but we need to acknowledge that disclosure may not be right for all people with dementia. There are circumstances when disclosing diagnosis will prove harmful and useless and where the benefits of disclosure cannot be achieved. The key to ensuring a correct decision with regard to disclosure will lie, as so many care options do, in knowing the individual.

Consideration should be given to whether knowing the diagnosis will make it easier for the person to cope with what is happening and whether they will realistically be able to use that knowledge to benefit from the identified advantages of disclosure. What the person is saying about what is happening to them can also aid the process of deciding to disclose diagnosis. Are they asking direct questions? Have they previously said that in the event of their contracting dementia or any serious illness they would not want to know? Consider also what the consequences of withholding the diagnosis might be.

There seems to be a difference in telling a person who is newly diagnosed with early stage dementia and informing someone who is moderately to severely affected by the disease. This is not to say that in all cases the person in the later stages should not be informed but that the onus is on whoever is disclosing to ensure appropriate support is in place in order that the advantages of disclosure can be realised. If this is not the case disclosure may at best be a wasted exercise and at worse abusive. What is clear is that further research is required to inform the process and the circumstances under which it is appropriate to withhold a diagnosis of dementia from the person with it.

Evidence for Practice

Is Disclosure Right for Everyone?

There is insufficient evidence about what people with dementia want with regard to disclosure

Older adult peer groups would want diagnosis to be disclosed if they developed dementia

The cognitive changes that are part of the dementia syndrome mean disclosure may not be right for everyone

One way forward is that disclosure be made to those able to benefit from the advantages of knowing what is wrong with them

There seems to be consensus that disclosure to people with early stage dementia is more desirable than disclosure to those in later stages

THE PROCESS OF DISCLOSURE

Once a diagnosis has been achieved and a decision taken to disclose to the person with dementia consideration needs to be given to the manner of disclosure. In a review of opinion and practice in disclosing a diagnosis of dementia Carpenter and Dave (2004) propose that 'sensitivity to individual differences may promote an optimal approach to disclosure'. This is true with regard to all aspects of disclosure: whether to disclose, who should disclose, what should be disclosed and when disclosure should be undertaken and how. The benefits to the client as well as the benefits for the professional will be that disclosure undertaken in an appropriate manner provides a foundation for the care relationship that is based on trust, fosters open and honest communication and establishes a plan of care from which to go forward.

As the coordinator of the diagnostic process the psychiatrist is the person most likely to disclose diagnosis. This may be true of the neurologist in the case of younger people with dementia. Given the hierarchy that persists in the public perception of things medical there is also an expectation on the part of most patients that the consultant as the senior member of the care team will impart the diagnosis. The support of other members of the specialist care team will be important in ensuring that the individual has access to pertinent information and services. Other members of the multidisciplinary team should develop their own skills in disclosure. Disclosing a diagnosis of any major illness is rarely a one-off event; it is a process and individuals will need a continuing supply of information relevant to their current situation. We have also seen that disclosing a diagnosis of dementia holds complications in that the individual may need to have the information disclosed on more than one occasion. The consultant may undertake the initial disclosure but members of the multidisciplinary team will need to be prepared to continue or repeat the process of disclosure.

The amount of information given at the point of disclosure should depend on a judgement of how much the individual wants to know and can cope with. Some people will want to know as much as possible straight away while others prefer information applicable to what is happening to them at that moment in time.

Several pieces of research into diagnosis disclosure raise the issue of language, the words professionals use when discussing 'dementia' with either carers or the individual with the disease. In order perhaps to soften the blow the word 'dementia' is frequently avoided and the issue of diagnosis is discussed in terms of 'memory difficulty' or 'confusion'. People with dementia already know they have difficulty remembering. What they need to know is that it is caused by dementia; they then need to know what dementia is, how they can expect it to affect their lives now and in the future and what help, treatment, advice and solutions can be offered in order that they can live their lives with the least disruption and best quality possible.

The forum of a multidisciplinary meeting where all professionals are available to answer the individual's questions may best facilitate the act of disclosure. However, many find entering a room filled with specialists daunting and considering the potentially shocking effect of the diagnosis individuals are likely to be in no fit state to either think of or pose the questions they want answers to. At a later stage ensuring access to the appropriate professional for information may prove vital to enable the person with dementia to discuss aspects of their experience, to have it explained to them and to allow them to consider possible avenues of action. It is rare for anyone to leave a doctor's meeting having recalled and understood all that has been said, so offering written information on dementia may be useful.

The act of disclosure is frequently undertaken within the clinical environment. Such areas are infrequently suitable for this purpose. Individuals may be one of several patients being seen during a consultant's clinic and once the information is given they may be expected to vacate the room for the next person to be seen.

Subjects in the study undertaken by Pratt and Wilkinson (2001) describe wanting disclosure to take place in a small, pleasant room. The force of receiving the diagnosis is enough to concentrate on without having to battle with an unpleasant environment. The environment should be in a place where other people cannot overhear and where the individual and their family can sit for a while following disclosure in order to begin to absorb the information that has been given. Offering a member of the care team to stay with them for a period of time underlines the gravity of what has been disclosed, affords an opportunity to ask questions and reinforces to the person with dementia that this is something they are likely to need time to come to terms with and help to live with.

Information from all sources, from people with dementia and from specialist workers, indicates that diagnosis should be achieved early. As discussed at the outset of this chapter, disclosure should be made as soon as possible so that the individual with dementia can take advantage of the information while still fairly fit. With regard to when during the week or day to disclose, it makes sense to avoid evenings and in particular a Friday evening, as most services for people with dementia are unavailable after 17.30 and at weekends (although this is changing) and individuals may have difficulty contacting appropriate people for information outside office hours.

Some preparation should be applied to the initial act of disclosure. The individual should ideally be invited to meet with the person undertaking disclosure and given the opportunity to decide who else is involved. It should be made explicit that they may bring someone with them if they wish. With regard to older people in particular research reflects that the majority of people want other family members to have information about what is happening to them (Sullivan et al. 2001).

The best way to deliver bad news is an area that the majority of health professionals will have had no formal training in. The syllabus for mental health nurse training, although concentrating on communication skills, does not include the practice of delivering diagnosis or other bad news. Barnet (2004) reports that since the 1990s communication skills training for medical undergraduates has become well established but practice in delivering bad news is still considered a skill to be learned on the job.

Communication skills are important in this area as they enable one to decide how to progress through the act of disclosure, interpreting not only what the patient says verbally but also what their nonverbal communication is conveying. First and foremost, during the act of disclosure it is the person with dementia who should be spoken to. This may seem obvious, but when the individual struggles to show understanding of what is said professionals have a tendency to turn to family and give them information, not infrequently, literally over the head of the person with dementia. This is no longer acceptable professional behaviour. Addressing the person with dementia will enable the person disclosing to establish what they already know about their difficulties or the tests they have had. This in turn will enable the professional to decide where to start the conversation.

The progress of the discussion should be at a pace acceptable to the person, with frequent checking of their understanding and continued wish for information. The process of disclosing a diagnosis should not be viewed as something that can be undertaken at a ten minute outpatient appointment. The person disclosing should be prepared for emotion to be expressed; anger, disbelief, distress and shock are not uncommon. The expressed emotion should not be ignored and appropriate comment reflecting empathy should be offered.

There is only so much that can be disclosed at the initial discussion but it is important that something positive be offered. Where a diagnosis with regard to what is causing the person's dementia has been established, the information discussed in Chapter 1 will be useful in advising on drug treatments and lifestyle changes as potential benefits to the person's condition.

Where the person disclosing the diagnosis feels they can offer nothing positive in the line of medical treatment the focus of the conclusion of the discussion should be around how the individual can be enabled to live with dementia, the services and the support available in learning to come to terms with dementia. Written information should be offered and contact points for local support groups, for example the Alzheimer's Society, made available. The person with dementia should be offered the opportunity to ask questions throughout the discussion, particularly when drawing the discussion to a close.

As the discussion closes it should be made clear what the next step is with regard to professional involvement for the person and those significant to them. It is at this point also that providing a private space for the person and those with them to compose themselves before they leave becomes important. Being able to offer such a facility enables the person making the disclosure to bring the meeting to an end but continue to acknowledge the impact of what has been discussed.

Evidence for Practice

The Process of Disclosure

When

As soon as possible after diagnosis

Not late afternoon or when services are likely to be closed

Who

Usually the consultant initially

All members of the multidisciplinary team (MDT) have a role

Where

A private room

How

Speak to the person with dementia

Ensure significant others are present if that is what the individual wants

Employ good communication skills

Allow time

Establish what the individual already knows

Establish and check regularly how much the individual wants to know

Regularly check understanding and allow an opportunity to question

Go at the individual's pace

Empathise with expressed emotion

Offer hope

Support verbal with written information

Establish the next step

Offer an opportunity to use a quiet period to absorb the information

Disclosure should be viewed as an ongoing process that may need to be repeated

For far too long providing the individual with an explanation for their change in cognition and functioning has been viewed as unnecessary. In the light of what we now understand about the person's experience of dementia, giving such an explanation is not only a right but for many a necessity, and from what we know about the individual's capacity to develop coping strategies in learning to live with dementia it is their right to receive a diagnosis sooner rather than later. The onus on professionals is that they develop ways of telling the person that they have dementia in a manner responsive to their individual needs and capabilities.

SUPPORT FOLLOWING DIAGNOSIS

Developing best practice in diagnosis disclosure is vital. Disclosing a diagnosis of dementia in a supportive manner is the first step in enabling the individual and those close to them to develop ways of living with dementia that enhance daily life quality. Providing appropriate support and follow-up should be the next step. If the aim of disclosure is to obtain the benefits thereof then it falls also within our remit to provide structures that support individuals with dementia in achieving the benefits of knowing they have dementia.

Support groups, outpatient follow-up, counselling, home visits by specialist workers, a coordinated package of care and information on new products, services and treatments are all part of the health and social care service package routinely offered to people with other debilitating and devastating diagnoses and there is no reason why there should be less of a service available for people with dementia. However, what is available for people with dementia is very variable and depends frequently on local issues, resources and indeed individual champions within localities. Thus in many parts of the country those in the early stages of dementia are likely to be given their diagnosis and followed up at outpatient appointments of six monthly or yearly intervals until their condition deteriorates such that they warrant an increase in service. While this might appear a reasonable use of precious resources it ignores the primary focus of early diagnosis and diagnosis disclosure – the drive to provide the individual with information that will empower and enable them to learn to live with dementia. Add to this the fact that research has shown (Yale 1995) that support in the early stages of dementia can delay the need for more intensive support at a later date and the need to offer support following diagnosis disclosure is clear.

Evidence for Practice

Support Following Diagnosis

It is important to provide support following diagnosis

Support will enable the individual to cope with the diagnosis, develop ways to live with dementia and obtain the benefits of the disclosure of diagnosis

Support groups, outpatient follow-up, counselling, home visits by specialist workers, a coordinated package of care, information on new products, services and treatments all constitute means by which people with dementia can be supported

---

SUPPORT GROUPS FOR PEOPLE DIAGNOSED WITH EARLY STAGE DEMENTIA

One avenue of practice that is engaging the interest of professionals as a tool to support people in the early stages of dementia and particularly following disclosure of diagnosis is the medium of support groups. The focus of support groups is to bring people with common experiences together. The function of such groups is to enable people to share their experiences, to provide understanding, information and support and to enable individuals to find new ways to cope with common problems. Support groups are frequently set up in response to the common experience of life changing events. As such they are an appropriate resource for people with dementia and particularly important for people newly diagnosed in the early stages of dementia.

Cheston *et al.* (2003) describe a project involving six psychotherapeutic groups set up in the south of England, each aiming to bring people with dementia together to discuss and share experiences. They found that levels of depression among participants declined during the course of the 10-week group programme and that individuals were able to come to terms with having dementia.

Yale (1995) describes support groups developed in the United States that aim, as Yale terms it, to address 'the blind spot' in dementia care that has left people with the disease no opportunity to react to or develop strategies with regard to living with dementia. Yale's groups grew out of a desire to provide a forum through which people with dementia who seek help can receive the help, as Yale states, 'in order to deal with their emotional reactions, problem-solve their current situations, and plan for the future'. We can therefore understand the potential power of support groups in enabling people with early stage dementia to attain the benefits of knowing their diagnosis.

In this country establishing support groups for people with dementia is a relatively new approach. Group work with people with dementia, other than activity based, has little foundation historically and people working in the care specialism are unlikely to have specialised group work skills. This has the potential to put people off developing such groups in their local area. What follows is a description of how to set up a support group for people with dementia. This process is based on the available research and my own clinical experience.

Many people with experience of working with people with early stage dementia have an ability, arguably the greatest skill, to communicate with people who have dementia. This is the ability to adjust to patterns and content of speech that are not always easy to follow, to understand what is being communicated, to use questions and prompts, to interpret and encourage and to empathise in order to help people with dementia to express their needs and emotions. Such skills are essential in a support group facilitator.

For those already communicating in a skilled way with people who have dementia the step to establishing successful support groups lies in being able to apply these skills to a group of people rather than on a one-to-one level. There is a need also to anticipate and be able to deal with the expression of deep emotion within a group setting. The information being discussed will be upsetting at times.

Together with skill in communication the group facilitator should have an extensive knowledge of dementia, in order that group participants can have answers to their questions. The optimum method of developing skill in running support groups is to observe someone else facilitating a group supported by someone with experience. Continued supervision for facilitators is vital in order to ensure that they are supported in delivering this service. There are also several key aspects that require consideration when establishing such groups.

Understanding of issues that will be pertinent to individuals with early stage dementia is one key as this will be the focus of the group's activity. Knowing what individuals are likely to want to discuss is essential. This will help the facilitators to draw up a programme that will constitute the format of the group.

It should be envisaged that the format will include discussion of treatment options, types of dementia and prognosis, common difficulties and shared solutions, how having dementia makes you feel, how it affects relationships and how individuals can help themselves. Addressing these topics within the group will provide the opportunity for people to start achieving the benefits of having their diagnosis. It is also probable that practical issues will need to be addressed, for example advice and education on financial planning and pursuing independent activity (including driving, where appropriate) and what resources are available within the local community. Having a set format for the activity of the group should be tempered by the ability on behalf of the facilitators to allow group participants to focus on what is most important to them. Apart from the experience and skill of the people who will facilitate the group another aspect key to success is the number of facilitators available to run the group. Each group should have a minimum of two workers. As one worker facilitates group discussion the other or others should be attentive to the behaviour of the group's participants and support them emotionally or enable them to join the discussion as appropriate. There is likely to be a variance in participants' ability to contribute verbally or express themselves and the facilitators have an important role in ensuring that all members are enabled to express themselves in a way that allows them to benefit from group processes. There will also be the occasion where, for any number of reasons, a group participant needs to leave the group, for example to use the toilet or if they have become unsettled. A lone facilitator cannot deal with such eventualities. It is also worth bearing in mind that having a minimum of facilitators will mean that the group will have to be cancelled in the event of a facilitator's unavailability. The number of available facilitators will have an impact on the size of the group, but considering the special needs of individuals with dementia with regard to communication a smaller group setting is beneficial. A group with as few as four and as many as twelve members can be successful, although the optimum number is probably eight. This generally ensures there are enough people to carry the conversation and include everyone.

The criteria for acceptance to the group and under what circumstances a participant might be excluded from the group need serious consideration. There should be an agreed understanding of what constitutes early stage dementia. Relevant considerations will include the individual's verbal ability, ability to recall their diagnosis, cognitive ability, support outside the group, how attendance would benefit the individual and, importantly, whether the individual wants to participate. Excluding an individual on the basis of any of the agreed criteria need not necessarily exclude them from the benefits of such support, but perhaps the support needs to be offered in a different way, for example on a one-to-one level or through the medium of memory support groups for individuals with more advanced dementia. Prior to starting the group facilitators should consider the individual make-up of participants and how this might impact on the way in which the group is conducted and what might be needed from facilitators in terms of language and understanding of cultural issues.

Further important considerations prior to the start of diagnosis support groups include the duration and frequency over which the group will run. Yale (1995) describes an evidence-based model running over eight weeks and lasting 90 minutes per week; Yale's model includes running parallel group sessions for carers to address their needs. I have experience of running diagnosis support groups within day services where a morning session of diagnosis support is followed by an afternoon group involving cognitive stimulation activity. Cognitive stimulation therapy is a method through which the individual strengthens their existing resources; one recent study by Knapp *et al.* (2006) found this work to be not only beneficial to the quality of life but as effective as antidementia drugs. Cognitive stimulation therapy is discussed further in Chapter 7.

There also need to be decisions on where the group will be held. Although this may be dependent on what is available, it is important to consider basic requirements such as size (will the group fit comfortably into the room allocated) and whether there are easily accessible toilets, tea-making facilities and space for individuals to spend time if they leave a session early. Can participants readily reach and access the venue?

Facilitators might also want to decide whether the group will be open or closed. An open group would mean that numbers could be consistent even if people dropped out; this might also be helpful if a waiting list was in operation. The advantage of a closed group would be that with membership static the individuals in the group might form closer bonds and feel safer in sharing personal information.

Consider also how participants will be recruited. It should be decided whether referrals will be required and if so from whom – psychiatrists, general practitioners (GPs) or the Alzheimer's Society for example.

There are many facets to establishing support groups for people newly diagnosed with early stage dementia and previous lack of experience might put some people off doing so. However, in common with people with any major diagnosis people with dementia deserve the opportunity to have needs for assistance, information and support catered for. Because people with dementia present us with complex considerations in establishing support groups there is no reason why we should not do so. Most of the salient points for consideration prior to running such a group are outlined above and the model presented by Yale (1995) in her book entitled *Developing Support Groups for Individuals with Early-Stage Alzheimer's Disease* is both evidence based and easy to replicate. The main considerations in setting up and running a support group are summarised below. A wider application in practice should engender further research and provide broader evidence through which we can improve our practice.

Evidence for Practice

Establishing Support Groups for People with Early Stage Dementia

What is needed from facilitators

Knowledge and experience of group work

Expert knowledge of dementia

Good communication skills

An understanding of the common life issues for people with early stage dementia

What is needed from individuals with dementia

A diagnosis of early stage dementia

Willingness to participate

Programme elements

Treatment options

Types of dementia and prognosis

Common difficulties and shared solutions

How dementia makes you feel

How dementia affects relationships

How individuals can help themselves

Practical issues

Group structure

Number of members

Duration and frequency

Open or closed

Venue

A room that will comfortably accommodate the number of people attending

Easy access for people with a physical disability

Access to housekeeping facilities

Recruitment

From outpatient clinic

GP referral

Self-referral

From other groups, such as the Alzheimer's Society

CONCLUSION

The unanimous calls for early diagnosis of dementia make sense only in a health care environment that uses the ability to diagnose early to the benefit of the individual with dementia. This involves not only informing the person that they have dementia but supporting them in coping with that information and in developing personal strategies that enable them to live the best quality of life that it is possible for them to live with dementia. At present our ability as a health community to diagnose dementia vastly outstrips our ability to disclose the diagnosis appropriately or to provide proper support where we do disclose. There should be urgency on the part of those of us who are members of this health community, psychiatrists, mental health nurses, social workers, occupational therapists and psychologists, to use the evidence, however sparse, to develop and share approaches that will lead to defined best practice sooner rather than later.

5 Perspectives on the Experience of Dementia

INTRODUCTION

This chapter examines what it is like to live with dementia and crucially how we can utilise the information given by people who have dementia to improve their experiences of living with dementia. We begin by looking at why the perspective of the person with dementia was for so long ignored and why and how we are now beginning to realise that personal awareness and experience is retained by the person throughout the course of their dementia. We examine what it is like to have dementia, using personal accounts, and the importance of using these accounts to inform care practice. The role of depression in dementia is considered. There is discussion also of the experiences of family members, the effect on family relationships and the emotional impact of living with someone who has dementia.

THE IGNORED EXPERIENCE OF DEMENTIA

Historically one of the key components of the approach to dementia care was a lack of understanding of what it is like to have dementia. There are many reasons why first-hand accounts of the experience of dementia have not been influential in developing care services. The consequences for people with dementia within the care system have been catastrophic. Cotrell and Schulz (1993) identified a lack of attention to what the person with dementia has to say, which reduces the person to 'an entity to be studied rather than someone who can directly contribute to an understanding of the illness and its course'.

The ability of someone with dementia to detail their perception fluently of what is happening to them is lost as the disease progresses. Language deteriorates and word finding becomes problematic. Other methods of communication that are easily inter-pretable by others become increasingly hard and by the time dementia has progressed to the middle stage the person has extreme difficulty expressing themselves. This difficulty with communication impairs the person's ability to portray themselves as individuals, to express what they are feeling or to detail what is good or bad in their lives. In the absence of any commentary that could be easily interpreted by carers the traditional response has been to *assume* that individuality is lost, that the person has no self-awareness and that they are thus not experiencing what is happening to and around them. It is this assumption that is directly responsible for the stagnation of the dementia care specialism and the reduction of the individual to the status of 'entity to be studied' rather than a contributory partner in the care process. It is this assumption that allowed Jacques as recently as 1992 to advise:

> Our feelings about what is good or humane for a severely demented patient cannot come from an understanding of what she feels as an individual, or of what she 'wants'. These concepts are meaningless and so any real understanding is impossible. At the final stages the patient may be assumed to have no real subjective awareness, no sense of self at all, and to be in this sense mentally 'dead'.

Jacques' comments are representative of traditionally accepted 'facts' about people with dementia and illustrate how a lack of research into psychosocial aspects of dementia has left the specialism reliant on 'facts' that are based on assumptions. This is no longer an acceptable basis from which to develop and deliver care. Indeed, we are just beginning to understand how detrimental an effect harbouring such beliefs has had and continues to have on the lives of people with dementia.

A further factor contributing to a lack of personal accounts of experience on the part of people with dementia was the lack of contact with service providers at the stage when the ability to describe that experience was intact. There can be no doubt that in the early stages of dementia the individual can more easily comment on their experience. However, prior to the advent of antidementia drugs it was not common practice for professional carers to have prolonged contact with people with early stage dementia. Therefore the window of opportunity – that time when the person could most easily convey experience – was the time they were least likely to have contact with professionals. By the time such contact was established the ability to convey experience in ways easily understood was seriously compromised. This led to overreliance on the perspective of family and informal carers, so it is *their* experience that has been relied upon extensively to inform practice development.

Even where the individual with dementia was obviously distressed and upset, feelings that might be reflected in shouting, continuous walking, aggression or withdrawal, this was most frequently attributed to dementia rather than a reasonable response by the individual to what was happening to and around them. Growing evidence of the effects of this disregard for the lived experience of dementia, particularly on the part of professional carers, has led to a realisation that we, as the previously acknowledged experts in dementia care, actually contributed to making the life quality of individuals with dementia poorer. In believing for so long that the individual was not aware of what was happening to them we have developed little understanding of what it is like to live with dementia. As a result empathy, arguably the key skill in mental health care, has been largely absent from care practice.

Carers have long understood that dementia was something they would not want to have themselves and *sympathy* has been an element of care. However, sympathy results largely in maternal caring approaches that are often patronising, disempowering and at worst abusive. Kitwood (1997) details some of these behaviours on the part of carers in his descriptions of a 'malignant social psychology'. He provides vivid descriptions of interactions between carers and individuals with dementia that reflect total disregard for the individual's abilities, dignity or self-esteem and that put the blame for inability squarely on the individual. Kitwood's observations were all the more significant because the majority of us working in 24-hour care settings recognised the scenarios he described and could provide similar scenarios directly from our own experience.

Empathy acknowledges the role of the sufferer and their experiences and gives them power within the care relationship. However, empathy is difficult to foster in an environment where people with dementia are believed to have no awareness or experience. The development of a concrete understanding of what it is like to have dementia can come only through listening to people with dementia who tell us what it is like to have dementia: how it disrupts their lives and relationships and how it impacts on their ability to demonstrate to those with whom they have contact and upon whom they are frequently dependent that they are worthwhile human beings.

The importance of the contribution of the individual with dementia cannot be underestimated. The services available for people with dementia must be directed at meeting their needs. This will only be achieved when those developing and providing services have a sound understanding of their needs, which in turn will only occur when service providers consult with people who have dementia. As we shall see, research is now providing evidence of retention of self-awareness throughout the course of dementia and evidence that persons with dementia retain the ability to comment on their experience, albeit in ways that require great skill to access. In the past consultation has not taken place because service providers believed that people with dementia were unable to be involved in such consultation. We are learning that this is not only possible but essential. The onus is on us as service providers to uncover, confirm and apply the results of such consultation. The repercussions of discounting the subjective experience of dementia are summarised below.

Evidence for Practice

The Repercussions of Discounting the Lived Experience of Dementia

Reduces the individual to an 'entity'

Encourages sympathy rather than empathy, leading to poor care practices

Leads to the development of practice that is not reliant on the expressed preferences of persons with dementia

Leads to distressed behaviour being interpreted as a symptom of illness

Denies the individual the opportunity to be a contributory partner in care

Disempowers people with dementia

EVIDENCE OF EXPERIENCE AND AWARENESS

Conventionally information about the lived experience of an individual with a particular illness or disease is taken directly from the person with the disease or illness. The medical profession and the health community have an interest in gathering such information from a research perspective and the world of the media has long reflected both the need of individuals to talk about what is happening to them and the curiosity of the general public in wanting to know what it is like to live and die with specific diseases. Detailing experience through books, magazine articles, television appearances, documentaries and film is commonplace. Such documentary evidence is useful in that it enables the health care community to develop a broad understanding of illness and facilitates a holistic approach to care rather than one based purely on medical signs and symptoms. The empathy engendered by such personal depiction of illness is also useful in mobilising understanding in carers and generating funds for research and development. Representation of what it is like to have dementia is undeniably sparse in comparison to many illnesses that afflict the population, for example cancer or even other mental illnesses such as depression. However, in this area also change is occurring. Keady (1996) identified the voice of people with dementia, as spoken through autobiographical works, as being the catalyst for much of the interest and subsequent research into the experience of dementia from the perspective of the person living with it. Examples include those of Davis (1989) and McGowin (1993), people living with dementia explaining dementia from their side, the things that happened prior to diagnosis, achieving the diagnosis and the struggle to come to terms with living with the diagnosis and through the telling making clear the emotional experience of that journey. The existence of such works challenged the long held belief that people with dementia were passive subjects of their condition; here were people with dementia responding to what was happening to them, obviously active and with awareness of the impact dementia was having on their existence.

From the perspective of wanting to share their experiences openly some people with dementia are overcoming the shame and embarrassment they feel in order to support others with dementia and to enable members of the public, particularly care service providers, to understand what it is like to live with dementia. The Internet is also being used as a means of communicating and sharing experiences of having dementia. For example, www.alzheimersforum.org, a website run by and for people with dementia, provides an opportunity for people with dementia and others to exchange information and experiences. It is one of several such forums and even a brief visit to these forums illustrates clearly that not only do people with dementia have self-awareness but they possess the ability to describe their experiences of living with dementia and can clearly express what they need from service providers.

The research and work of early proponents of exposing the voice of people with dementia such as Kitwood (1997), Goldsmith (1996) and Keady and Nolan (1994) led the way in showing that the voice of subjective experience *is* there but considerable skill may be required to expose that voice. Although it may be true that people with early stage dementia are most articulate in their ability to tell what it is like to have dementia, there is research that supports the ability of people in the later stages of dementia to display an appreciation of their experience. Miesen (1997) cites research and clinical observations that have shown that people with Alzheimer's disease still respond to their illness long after insight into the illness has disappeared. Tappen *et al.* (1999) also found evidence suggesting that individuals with Alzheimer's disease in the middle to late stages retain an awareness of self and changes in their cognition and warn against a failure to recognise this as leading to care that is task orientated and poor in therapeutic intervention. Ostwald *et al.* (2002) provide evidence that people with dementia with mini-mental state results (Folstein *et al.* 1975) ranging from 5 to 28 were able to comment on their experience. Sabat (2002) confirmed that a sense of self persists in individuals with moderate to severe dementia and further that loss or potential loss of an individual's social persona is more likely a result of healthy people reducing the status of the individual to being a burden or being dysfunctional rather than a result of dementia.

Our current understanding of what it is like to have dementia is beginning to be framed by research that consults with people who have dementia. This research is open to criticism in that sample groups are often small, thus generating concern about applying the results to a larger population. However, given that this field of research is on the whole less than 15 years old and that there are specific difficulties associated with involving people with dementia in research, the aspect to celebrate is that the body of research is growing, it is informing practice and it is enabling us to make life better for people with dementia.

Developing understanding of the experience of dementia from the individual's perspective is enabling us to identify the common experiences that face the majority of people with dementia. By so doing we are able to develop services that specifically address collective needs. An example of this is how by listening to people with dementia carers came to appreciate the immense stress of receiving a diagnosis of dementia. This is leading to the development of support groups for people newly diagnosed with early stage dementia. Once services are in place the experience of those using the service will facilitate evaluation of that service. Thus we know from reports of the personal experiences of people using support groups that they are successful in helping people to begin to cope with diagnosis (Yale 1995). There is now significant evidence, from research and practice and from the mouths of people with dementia, that awareness of self and an appreciation of what is happening to and around the person with dementia are retained by the person throughout the progress of dementia.

People with dementia themselves are beginning to speak out through the medium of books, involvement in research, by speaking at conferences and by exchanging experiences in chat rooms set up for that purpose. The onus is on us as carers to support individuals in expressing what it is like to have dementia and to ensure that information is used to influence service development. Although historically the role of the individual with dementia in voicing their experiences has been denied and the results have been detrimental to care practices and the experience of care, we now have evidence that the person with dementia can experience and can comment on that experience. The skill for carers lies in developing ways to access and integrate that experience into practice.

Evidence for Practice

The Significance of the Reported Experience of Dementia

Information on what it is like to live with dementia can broaden our understanding of dementia and promote a holistic approach to care

Research, personal narrative and media portrayal have provided evidence that awareness of self and the ability to comment on personal experience is retained in people with dementia even where dementia is severe

Acknowledging the experience of the person with dementia engenders empathy in carers

Information on the lived experience of dementia enables the development and evaluation of services appropriate to the needs of people with dementia

---

WHAT IS IT LIKE TO LIVE WITH DEMENTIA?

There can be little doubt that receiving a diagnosis of Alzheimer's disease or any other type of dementia is devastating to the individual and those close to them. Information widely available through the media means that significant numbers receiving the diagnosis will understand immediately that this diagnosis has the potential to alter their lives extensively and that the chances of a cure are remote. Research identifies several themes in regard to individuals' reported experiences of having dementia. Ostwald *et al.* (2002) found the primary experience is one of loss – loss of ability or loss of something that the individual has prior to developing dementia but no longer has as a result of now having dementia. Ostwald *et al.* found that people reported loss of the ability to remember, to initiate conversation, to think or control situations and even to remain in contact with reality. They were able to identify these themes consistently among the study subjects, regardless of the severity of dementia the person was experiencing.

Further, Ostwald *et al.* identified common emotional responses, including concern about family and being a burden, sadness, embarrassment about memory loss, fear, uncertainty and anger. However, the findings were not all negative: optimism, love, appreciation and satisfaction were also themes identified in the study and people described strategies they employed in order to cope with what they were experiencing. Strategies included cognitive, social and behavioural methods of managing what was happening to them.

In his written narrative on living with dementia Cary Smith Henderson (1998) recorded his experiences and feelings in an effort to provide a map for others with dementia to aid their understanding of what is likely to happen to them. His observations echo those of individuals in the Ostwald *et al.* study. He describes difficulties in his thinking, difficulty conversing and reading, problems with remembering and the loss of employment as dementia made it impossible for him to pursue his career in academia. He describes feeling a sense of shame and uselessness together with anger and frustration. He remarks, 'I do sincerely miss the things I used to have', underlining the sense of loss he feels.

In common with Ostwald's subjects Smith Henderson was also able to find positive experiences, acknowledging that at the point of diagnosis he and his wife were absolutely sure that everything was over, but that he learned to cope and indeed to take joy from things, like the company of his dog, watching birds in the garden and listening to music.

A study by Braudy Harris (2002) of the experiences of younger people with dementia reveals slightly different themes. Perhaps not surprisingly younger people found that they had great difficulty obtaining a diagnosis; dementia is largely perceived as a disorder of old age and atypical dementias more prevalent in individuals under the age of 65 and are thus more difficult to diagnose. Individuals also expressed distress at loss of self-esteem and changes in their perceptions of themselves as change in their abilities occurred as a result of dementia, for example having to stop work or give up driving. Change in roles and relationships were also issues. Younger people are more likely to hold multiple roles within the family, parent, spouse, sibling and child, and the balance within these relationships is significantly altered by dementia. Two of the study subjects lived with parents, several others with children upon whom they were increasingly dependent. One woman in her 40s commented on the difficulty she had remembering to collect her child from school, 'My memory is so bad that my youngest daughter would sometimes write her name all over my hand so that I wouldn't forget, and not pick her up.' The same woman concludes on her relationship with her husband: 'It is hard to believe you are a person who would be wanted when you are nothing like the person your spouse married.' The majority of individuals in Braudy Harris' study were very aware of what was happening to them and their families. One woman explains: 'I can handle that I will lose my life, but that my children's mother will die and leave them is unbearable to me.' Having to give up work and abandon careers potentially at their height was another issue for younger persons with dementia, together with the financial strain this puts on their families. One woman in the study expressed distress at having her children's college fund spent instead on care for her.

The fact that dementia has the effect of isolating people and making them feel marginalised is frequently commented upon and for younger people there is the added isolation of suffering from what is perceived as an old persons' illness. Another issue raised in the study was that of being a burden at an early age. In today's Western society independence is highly prized, but there is an expectation that with old age some level of dependency is inevitable. To have to be subject to such dependency at a younger age increases the stress for the person with dementia and indeed those upon whom they are dependent. Unsurprisingly boredom and loss of occupation were identified as issues for younger adults with dementia. One woman explains: 'It's a long, long day so I try to keep myself busy, but I mean you can only clean your house so much.' The Braudy Harris study demonstrates that having dementia at a younger age presents the individual with different challenges. However, what remains consistent in the experience of both younger and older adults with dementia is the sense of loss.

Kitwood (1997) recognised the themes of loss brought about by dementia and identified that the experience of living with dementia was compatible with the process of grief. As personal resources are increasingly lost due to dementia emotional responses on the part of the individual experiencing those losses are frequently grief responses, including denial, anger and depression. Kitwood (1997) cautioned that there is a risk for the person with dementia of becoming stuck in the depression stage, preventing the completion of the grief process. This means that the individual does not progress from depression to accepting what is happening and completing the cycle by achieving a reconstruction of life with dementia. Coping with the life changing difficulties that dementia brings is difficult enough, but to struggle to do so in the face of a depressive illness must be nearly impossible. Professionals are beginning to realise that depression is far from rare in people who also have dementia and they must bring to their practice a habit of not only assessing for depression but also seeking treatment where it is confirmed.

What is abundantly clear is that living with dementia is largely a traumatic experience, an experience the person has to come to terms with while struggling with increasingly reduced cognitive ability, being potentially consumed with the actuality of losing the strengths of personal ability they have developed through their lives and against a background of changing family relationships and feelings of grief. What is also emerging is that in spite of this trauma people with dementia do find strategies to enable them to live with dementia and do find positive aspects in new ways of living.

Evidence for Practice

What Is It Like to Live with Dementia?

The overriding experience of people with dementia is one of loss

Individuals frequently experience a grief reaction as a result of multiple losses

Losses include memory, control over thought processes, independence, ability to initiate conversation, ability to retain contact with reality

This grief process may stall at the depression stage, thus preventing individuals from progressing to the acceptance and reconstruction stages

The experience for younger people diagnosed with dementia is distinct in some ways from the experience for older adults

Not all experiences of living with dementia are negative and individuals do develop coping strategies

DEPRESSION IN DEMENTIA

There has been a growing recognition of depression in people who have dementia over the past 10 years. Draper (1999) identifies that for many years the focus of attention on depression in people who presented with symptoms of cognitive impairment was on differentiating between dementia and severe depression which might be misdiagnosed as dementia, so-called pseudo-dementia. Where a definite diagnosis of dementia was established, interest in identifying or treating depressive symptoms was largely lost. Draper also identifies the difficulties in accurately diagnosing depression in dementia due to the overlap in symptoms, including apathy, sleep disturbances, changes in appetite, concentration and psychomotor performance, loss of interests and social withdrawal, self-neglect and anxiety. The traditional response to symptoms of depression found in people who have dementia has been to accept it as symptomatic of dementia and thus not requiring treatment. This accounts, says Draper, for the disparity in figures given for the prevalence of depression in dementia throughout the literature, where figures range from 0 to 86 % of people with dementia who also have depression.

If, as Kitwood identifies, depression occurs as part of a grief reaction to the experience of dementia and if it prevents people with dementia from potentially coming to terms with what is happening to them and moving on from there, then identifying and treating the depression becomes very important indeed. Some studies suggest that depression is a greater risk in vascular dementia and Lewy body dementia, but it has been identified in all types of dementia. Those who have previously suffered depression may also be more susceptible to developing depression with dementia. Overstall (2005) suggests that depression in Alzheimer's disease may be one of the most common mood disorders in all older adults. There is certainly enough evidence about the incidence of depression in dementia for depression to be investigated, particularly where the individual experiences change in mood or behaviour.

Depression has been found to occur at any stage of dementia and increasing the awareness of those around the individual about how depression may be manifest in dementia is important. Changes in mood and behaviour can indicate the presence of depression. Changes in behaviour may include refusing to eat, aggression, agitation or withdrawal of cooperation. Of course other events such as infective illness may also account for changes in behaviour, making a definitive diagnosis difficult. There are specific tools available to aid diagnosis of depression in dementia, the Cornell scale (Alexopoulos *et al.* 1988) being one, but information from all sources, the individual themselves, family and other carers and observation of behaviour, should inform the diagnostic process. Where doubt exists it is not unreasonable to treat for depression in the hope of eliciting some improvement.

Treatment for depression in people with dementia ranges from psychotherapeutic approaches, which are to a large extent dependent on cognition and insight on the part of the individual, to antidepressant medication and, in extreme cases, to electroconvulsive therapy. However, serious consideration should be given to the individual's social environment and to improving stimulation and social engagement. This is particularly relevant where the individual is living alone and socially isolated or living in 24-hour care, where social isolation may be even more pronounced. Too frequently in 24-hour care settings the recipient of care can see others and hear others but is not offered enough opportunity to engage in social relationships that acknowledge their worth or confirm that they have a social status. As we have already seen, a sense of self is threatened by the behaviour of healthy people treating people with dementia as a burden or as being dysfunctional (Sabat 2002). There are many causes of depression in dementia; social isolation compounded by repeated denial on the part of others that the individual is worthy of social attention, if not a causal factor of depression, certainly contributes to its persistence. Therefore the importance of creating opportunities for social engagement with people with dementia and developing skills that enable that communication to be meaningful cannot be overemphasised.

The experience of depression has been found to exacerbate disability in people with dementia and to add to the burden of care, both physically and emotionally. The improvement in life quality that treating depression can bring is potentially no different in people with dementia than in people without dementia. Feelings of hopelessness, helplessness, guilt, apathy and overwhelming sadness, including wishes for death or suicidal thoughts, have no less impact on people with dementia than without. Ignoring depression or refusing to provide treatment on the basis of the individual having dementia is no longer acceptable care practice.

Evidence for Practice

Depression and Dementia

Depression can affect individuals with any type of dementia

Depression can occur at any stage of an individual's dementia

Depression can exacerbate dementia

Changes in mood and behaviour of the individual may signify the presence of depression

Information from all sources is required to make an accurate diagnosis, the person themselves, family and carers

A diagnosis of dementia should not preclude treatment of depression

Treatments include psychotherapeutic approaches, antidepressant medication and in extreme cases electroconvulsive treatment

Concentrating on the individual's social environment and improving stimulation may be the most effective treatment

USING THE EXPERIENCE OF DEMENTIA
TO INFORM PRACTICE

As we have already seen, developing an appreciation of what it is like to live with dementia can broaden our understanding of the syndrome and enable empathy to be fostered in carers. The information provided by people with dementia will only be of real value if, in partnership with people who have dementia, we develop ways of using that information to bring positive change to care practice and service provision. There are two primary methods of utilising information gained and both rely on our acknowledgement of people with dementia not only as partners in care but as experts on what it is like to live with dementia. Firstly, we can use research to canvas the opinions of groups of people with dementia, obtain details on common experiences and extrapolate this information to develop frameworks around which we can build service models to meet the needs of the majority. Secondly, we can attend to individuals' opinions on their experiences of their physical and psychosocial environment to enable attention to be paid to individual needs so that the service designed to meet the needs of the majority can be adapted to suit the individual. Used in tandem, these methods have the potential to improve significantly the services offered and to address poor practice.

As an example we can illustrate the potential importance of the former by looking at the framework first described by Keady and Nolan in 1994 to explain the experience of dementia from a temporal perspective. This framework was later refined and confirmed through direct consultation with people with dementia. Keady (1996) describes nine stages that the individual with dementia moves through from the point of realising that something is not quite right to dying with dementia. The importance of such a framework is that it enables us to have a better understanding of the needs of people at any stage of dementia. This allows decisions to be made about what is appropriate in terms of services and the way services are delivered.

Keady and Nolan identify the process as beginning prior to diagnosis, at the point when the individual first realises that they are experiencing memory lapses. This is termed 'slipping'. At this stage the individual rationalises what is happening to them, and they may believe that such memory lapses are normal for their age. As dementia progresses and the lapses become more frequent it becomes more difficult for the individual to rationalise what is happening. This stage, termed 'suspecting', is when the person realises that something is definitely wrong. The response to this realisation is to hide difficulties; this is a conscious decision by the person with dementia, which Keady and Nolan term 'covering up'. The next stage involves the person sharing concerns with others, generally someone close to them, termed 'revealing'. 'Confirming' is the stage when outside help is sought and diagnosis reached. Following confirmation of diagnosis the person adapts to their situation by developing coping strategies; this stage is referred to as 'maximizing'. 'Disorganization' follows, when the person experiences loss of ability and decline in awareness, which is followed by 'decline', a period when care is increasingly necessary. The final stage then is 'death'.

This framework allows us to understand that what people with dementia need at the early stage of dementia is quite different from what they are likely to require as dementia progresses. For example, we can consider that general education about memory loss in relation to age might prompt people to seek clarification on the nature of their memory deficits sooner, or that by tackling stigma attached to having dementia we might enable people at the suspecting stage to seek early diagnosis. Recognition that individuals adopt coping mechanisms to enable them to live with dementia opens up the prospect of being able to define services that support the development of coping strategies that help individuals to live more positively with dementia.

Conducting research with people with dementia will contribute to establishing frameworks to aid our understanding of dementia. Keady and Nolan's framework, as an example, explains the experience of dementia as a series of stages through which the individual passes as dementia progresses. This enables services to be designed congruent to the needs of people at various stages of experiencing dementia. Through such frameworks service models and care pathways can be designed and shared. Once models of care and pathways have been designed and implemented, we then need to ensure that what we have developed to suit the needs of the majority is appropriate for the individual – one size is unlikely to fit all. We need to have approaches that enable us to understand when what we are doing with, to or for the individual is not what they want. In effect we need to be able to access the experience of the individual in order to fine-tune our approaches to ensure that the experience is positive for them.

This is certainly easier when people are in the earlier stages of dementia and where verbal communication is relatively intact, but greater skill and use of other methods will be needed when the communication process becomes more difficult. Chapter 6 concentrates on the needs of people with dementia with regard to communication, but several commentators offer different ways of gaining information about the person's perspective.

Kitwood (1997), as we saw in Chapter 3, suggests seven routes of access to enhance our appreciation of the subjective experience of dementia. These methods of communication, observation and interaction represent ways in which we can gather information about the individual's perception of what is happening to and around them. Cheston (1996) points to the use of metaphors, which he (and other commentators) states are used by people with dementia to convey their emotional experience. He suggests that in recounting past events people with dementia may be giving a clear indication of their present emotions; people with dementia often speak through metaphors relating past events to describe their present experience. As a practice example, Cheston describes a man who spoke about his experiences during the War and his struggle to overcome vegetation in the jungle. Cheston interpreted this as a comment by the man on his current experience of struggling with his neurological deterioration which resulted from dementia. Though accepting accounts of past events and the emotions attached to that as a metaphorical way of expressing current emotions is difficult to evidence, there is significant acceptance of this theory by clinicians. Killick (2005) also provides accounts of the use of metaphors by persons with dementia and how the medium of poetry can be used to gain greater insight into what an individual is experiencing.

Kitwood (1997) states it is important to listen to people in the course of everyday life. The individual's conversation may be disjointed and words confused but with careful attention meaning can be gleaned that reflects the person's experience. In order to be effective the listener must be aware of the wider context of the person's life and experience, because the more we know about someone the greater the chance we have of understanding what they are communicating. Kitwood also proposed that we learn from the individual's behaviour and actions; even someone with advanced dementia will continue to use whatever ability remains with them to express themselves. This may be repetitive motion, rocking, rubbing or aggressive behaviour but, Kitwood cautions, such behaviour may be the person's 'last desperate bid to remain psychologically alive'. Indeed, it may be their last desperate bid to tell us about their experience of life and how they experience our behaviour and the environment they are living in. The onus is upon us to recognise such behaviour as a legitimate attempt to comment on what life is like for them and to respond or attempt a series of responses to comfort the individual and interpret their needs.

Kitwood was also instrumental in developing dementia care mapping (DCM), an audit tool developed primarily as a tool to improve standards of person centred care. DCM is an audit tool that involves observing individuals with dementia closely for long periods of time and making judgements on their experience of what happens to and around them. The process offers an invaluable opportunity to access the person's experience of what happens in their lives. In particular, as Brooker (2002) identifies, DCM can interpret the communication of people with dementia when they are distressed. This can greatly assist us in identifying aspects of care that have a negative impact on the individual, giving us the opportunity to change or avoid whatever it is in the psychosocial environment that is causing the distress. Equally, DCM enables clinicians to pinpoint aspects of care that the individual experiences in a positive way, allowing carers to ensure that the opportunity for positive experiences is increased.

Evidence for Practice

Using the Experience of the Person with Dementia

Applying the experience of dementia to care practice will broaden understanding, generate empathy and bring positive changes

People with dementia must be accepted as experts on what it is like to experience dementia and as key partners in developing and evaluating services

Research can help the development of frameworks to meet the needs of various groups of individuals living with dementia

Developing methods of discussing and observing the effects of care delivered through the frameworks will enable the needs of individuals to be addressed

Methods of accessing the experience of dementia are not exhausted when verbal communication becomes difficult, but include interpreting impaired communication and observing the behaviour of individuals

We are gradually building a quite different picture of dementia than that available in the literature 20 years ago. Within this picture the person with dementia is at the foreground, recognised as a feeling, thinking individual to whom traumatic changes are occurring but who retains the ability to tell others what this feels like. It is important that we use the tools available to continue to access the experience of individuals living with dementia effectively, with the goal of working in partnership so that they can be the ones whose experience and opinions grow, shape, develop and evaluate the services and care offered to them.

It is vital that we understand that it is no longer appropriate for those who do not have dementia to decide what people with dementia want or need and design services on that basis or to make assumptions about how an individual with dementia may be experiencing those services. Whether our practice takes us into the realms of research and focuses on answering specific questions or concentrates on day-to-day support for those living with dementia, we now know that it is possible for us to consult with and to utilise reported experience to empower people with dementia in improving their lives. The ability to tap into experience will facilitate our ability to change behaviour on our part and to alter environments within which we expect people with dementia to live. The goal of this activity must remain the improvement of life with dementia.

LIVING WITH SOMEONE WITH DEMENTIA

Discourse on dementia is littered with descriptions that portray those afflicted as problematic, stigmatised and impaired, degenerating cognitively and challenging in respect of their behaviour. Information from demographics describes dementia in terms of creating an impending epidemic and political strategy which, although occasionally couched in kinder terms, cannot help but refer to the *burden* created by people with dementia. This burden refers largely to the economic drain on health resources that people with dementia are perceived as being responsible for. With the cost of care rising steeply in relation to the severity of disease and the most expensive form of care being 24-hour institutional care, it is politically expedient to ensure that people requiring care remain in their own homes with care provided by their families for as long as possible. Fortunately the majority of people with dementia and their carers want the person with dementia to remain at home. The result, however, is that the true bearers of burden are the families of people with dementia, spouse, children and significant others, who with minimal physical, psychological and financial support attempt to manage the needs of the person they are caring for while struggling to maintain their own equilibrium. There is an expectation that individuals in these relationships will naturally assume the caring role and it is rare, particularly at the point of diagnosis, that any alternative is offered to the prospective caregiver. It is estimated that 80 % of the support required by older people is provided by the family (Walker 1995). The effects of caring on the caregiver are well documented and the cost of caring can be measured not only in monetary terms but in terms of the psychological and physical health of the carer. The effects are primarily negative.

Many carers have to reduce hours of paid employment significantly or cease paid work altogether in order to devote time to caring. This not only affects the weekly income but can impact on future pension or career opportunities. O'Shea (2003) found, in a study of carers in Ireland, that not only did two-thirds of carers in paid employment have to make adjustments to their working lives to facilitate caring but that the average cost in terms of loss of wages was more than £150 per week. Further financial pressure results where extra assistance in the form of private home care is required or aids to assist the care process are needed, for example drugs or incontinence pads. The financial strain of caring thus comes from two sources: the reduced opportunity to earn money and increased demands on finances available. Schulz *et al.* (1995), in reviewing dementia caregiving literature, report that psychiatric morbidity in carers is linked to income and that worry about money adds to the emotional strain. The psychological cost of undertaking a caregiver role is significant. Livingston *et al.* (1996) found that for carers of people with dementia the risks for both depression and anxiety are high. In a review of the literature concerning caregivers of people with dementia in 1995, Schulz *et al.*, found similarly that virtually all the studies reported raised levels of depression and anxiety in caregivers; indeed, in studies where diagnostic interviews were used high rates of *clinical* depression and anxiety were found. In 1999 Ory *et al.* comparing dementia and nondementia caregivers, found that all the negative aspects associated with the caregiver role had a higher impact on the individuals providing care for people with dementia. These include caregiver strain, reduction in time spent in paid employment or cessation of paid employment, physical and mental health problems, reduction in leisure time, reduction in time spent with other family members and conflict within the family.

Together with the psychological effects of caring, the carer is forced to cope with the changes that dementia initiates in the person and the changes in the relationship they previously had with that person. Loss is again a central theme – loss of intimacy, communication, control, roles and relationships. Adams and Sanders (2004) confirm that 'grief reactions and intense feelings of loss are not abnormal occurrences in caregivers of individuals with Alzheimer's disease'. That the physical health of carers is at a higher risk than noncarers is also confirmed by the evidence. Unsurprisingly, physical exhaustion and fatigue are reported by caregivers and increased susceptibility to illness and the use of medications together with self-reports of poor physical health are also found. Indeed, Schulz and Beach (1999) reported that care providers were at a significantly increased risk of death compared with noncaregivers.

The cost in terms of time spent caring is also significant, O'Shea (2003) reports carers spending up to 12 hours per day in caring and Max *et al.* (1995) found that of the 70 hours per week care that was needed 62 hours were provided by the main caregiver. The subjects of O'Shea's study were clear that this was significantly more time than they wanted to spend undertaking care and indeed other studies have highlighted the relentless nature of caring and the adverse effects this has on all areas of life. Svanström and Dahlberg (2004) describe how the lives of couples where one has dementia come to revolve around the dementia. Their actions are controlled by the effects of the disease, with the healthy partner taking more and more responsibility for day-to-day life and where planning for the future becomes impossible, other than the healthy spouse knowing that they will not cope for ever. When so much time is taken up providing care, the opportunity to carry on with accustomed routines of living, working, socialising, sustaining family and other relationships, planning for the future or setting even short term goals becomes unrealistic.

What we must always come back to is answering the question: 'How does the evidence enable a change in practice to benefit people living with dementia?' From the perspectives of carers much of the research leads us to an examination of the effects of providing care for people with dementia and how we can influence the factors contributing to the negative effects of caring to reduce the burden. With such an outcome in mind one area of interest is looking at determining the differences between caregivers who cope well and those who cope less well. Once the behaviour and approach of carers who cope well is described the aim is to teach others to adopt more positive approaches.

For example, a study by McClendon et al. (2004) suggests that interventions aimed at enhancing caregiver coping skills, focusing on problem solving and acceptance coping may benefit both carer and the care recipient. Almberg et al. (1997) also identified different strategies adopted by carers that had an impact on the levels of strain and burn-out they experienced. They found that a group of caregivers who used an emotion-focused strategy, including worrying, grieving and self-accusation, and who resorted to wishful thinking and stoicism experienced burn-out whereas those who adopted a more problem-focused strategy, including confronting the problem and seeking information and support, did not experience burn-out.

Approaches that address the caregiver experience in terms of burden and stress have been criticised by some commentators (Myers 2003), as they concentrate once again on the negative aspects of dementia and lead to interventions based on a medical model of care. Nolan et al. (2002) discuss the problems associated with concentrating efforts on reducing carer burden and conclude that despite a plethora of research on strategies aimed at reducing that burden little evidence of the effectiveness of such interventions is available. We could conclude therefore that despite significant information about the nature of caregiver burden there is little we can do to influence a reduction in that burden. It could also be concluded that the focus of research on the experience of carers that concentrates exclusively on the burden of the caring role is too narrow and that there are more factors involved in the caregiving relationship than what happens to the caregiver. Approaching carer's needs purely from the perspective of *burden* raises at least two major concerns: firstly, it ignores any positive outcomes to the caring role that might be influenced to improve life quality and, secondly, it addresses the needs of carers in isolation from the needs of the person with dementia.

Tarlow *et al.* (2004) identify that care giving can be a positive experience. Their study revealed that carers take satisfaction from feeling needed and useful and that caring made them feel good about themselves. This satisfaction is dependent on factors such as the prior relationship between the carer and the person with dementia, the carer being satisfied with the level of social support they receive and the use of problem-solving coping strategies on the part of the carer. Older carers and those in better physical health were also found to be more satisfied undertaking the caring role. Being able to identify positive aspects associated with care giving should enable support to be targeted at enhancing satisfaction for the caregiver.

To date the needs of the carer have largely been approached as distinct from the needs of the person with dementia. As a simple example, consider the carer who lacks sleep and rest because the behaviour of the person with dementia does not allow for sleep at night time. Addressing the needs of the carer, the solution lies in promoting night time sleeping in the person with dementia, which invariably involves the use of medication for the person with dementia. The outcome for the carer may be an increased chance of night time sleep, but this approach does not address the needs of the individual with dementia. In reality the carer may also reject such intervention as being unsatisfactory for the person they care for.

There is a requirement that research now considers the needs of people with dementia and their carers as a whole. There are a multitude of complex factors impacting on the caring situation. Some of these factors will relate to the individual with dementia, how they experience and express their needs, and some will be associated with the family, and in particular the main carer, and their satisfaction in and ability to provide appropriate care. In turn these factors will be influenced by the nature of the prior and current relationship between those involved. The reality is that these complex factors are interdependent and interrelated and attempting to unpick one from the other in order to achieve positive outcomes for people with dementia and those who care for them is unrealistic. Unfortunately, it is what service providers have been trying to do for many years.

The outcome of service providers' input should not be measured in terms of carer burden or in terms of how long and cheaply we can sustain the person with dementia at home. Rather we should concentrate on outcomes that seek to improve the quality of life of people with dementia and their carers, outcomes that acknowledge the range and expertise of existing skills in carers and that support the caring role by empowering both carer and cared for. This will involve working with and consulting those in the caring relationship. We are beginning to do this in other areas of dementia care and need to transfer the skills we are utilising to this area. It is also likely that some of the strategies we have developed thus far in support of the caring role, counselling, education and physical assistance, will continue to be important. As Nolan *et al.* (2002) identify: 'The most potent way of influencing the consequences of Alzheimer's disease will be to shape the support given to people with dementia and their carers.' There is a requirement that this shaping is influenced by the opinions and experiences of people who live day to day with dementia – the person with it and their carer. It is vital we direct research to the appropriate outcomes in order to develop suitable services; there are only so many resources available from health, social and voluntary services to deliver these approaches, so in effect we have to make the best of what we have. If we remain ignorant of the true needs of the caring relationship and those in it we can only continue to deliver guessed rather than best practice.

Evidence for Practice

The Carer's Experience

People with dementia, their carers and other key stakeholders want people with dementia to remain within their own home; the support systems we develop will be vital in ensuring this happens

Caring for someone with dementia impacts on the carer's psychological, social, physical and financial well-being

Carers of people with dementia are at increased risk of depression and anxiety

Research to date has concentrated on the 'burden' carers carry and intervention is designed to help carers cope with this burden

Targeting intervention purely on the carer ignores the needs of the person with dementia and the wider context of the caring relationship

More research targeting different outcomes is required to design appropriate support for the caring relationship

Consultation with people living with dementia, sufferers, carers and other family members, must inform the developmental process

---

CHILDREN LIVING WITH DEMENTIA

Adult caregivers are not the only people who have their lives disrupted by dementia. Considering the proportion of the population living with dementia we can appreciate the numbers of children and teenagers whose lives are transformed as parent, grandparent or greatgrandparent succumbs to the disease. The impact on their lives and the disruptions to relationships should not be ignored. Research into the effects of dementia on the lives of children and teenagers is sparse, which may mean that the needs of younger people are overlooked and that specific strategies to address their needs are underdeveloped.

Coming to terms with dementia within the family is difficult enough for an adult who may have access to professional or informal support and information from a multitude of sources. It is rarer for younger people to have access to such support or to be offered information, and it may also be difficult for them to understand explanations that are given about changes in behaviour or the ability of a family member with dementia. Indeed, in an effort to protect children from the harsh reality of this progressive syndrome adults may avoid talking to younger family members about what is happening.

In order to appreciate the younger person's perspective on living with dementia we need to consider several factors and their emotional and social impact. This includes not only changes to the person with dementia but also changes in those caring and who also have responsibility for younger family members and also the manner in which these changes alter family life and routines.

There may be changes in the relationship between the child and the person with dementia; this is compounded where the person with dementia is the child's main carer. The person with dementia may be unable to sustain previous levels of communication or maintain understanding of the needs of the younger person. Where hallucinations are a feature of dementia the child may be frightened or find the older person's behaviour a source of ridicule. Circumstances where the person with dementia forgets the name of the child or uses the wrong name can also be upsetting for the child. Braudy Harris (2002) provides examples of children trying to cope with the advent of dementia. The little girl writing on her mother's hand to ensure she remembers to pick her up has already been mentioned. That mother identifies that while outsiders may have thought using outside help was the solution to her inabilities they failed to recognise the emotional impact on her children of others undertaking their mother's role or the fear that losing abilities and the prospect of her early death generated in her children. Future research will undoubtedly reflect that having a parent with dementia as a young child or adolescent creates different needs from those identified in grown-up children.

Changes in other relationships may also disrupt the child's life. We have already seen how stressful and time consuming the role of caregiver can be. Children may struggle to understand and cope not only with changes to the person with dementia but changes in the mood and behaviour of family members who are caregivers for the person with dementia. Time and attention that was previously available for the younger family member may be lost.

All of these changes serve to disrupt accustomed routines within the home. The effects on children and adolescents should not be underestimated and care should be taken not to exacerbate the situation by presuming the younger person does not understand or notice what is happening. A lack of information may lead the child to worry that they are somehow to blame for what is happening or that they may catch dementia themselves.

Common emotional experiences may include jealousy and resentment as time and attention are focused away from the child, guilt as in the absence of any alternative explanation the child may presume they are to blame, and embarrassment about the behaviour of the older person, which may lead to the adolescent reducing social contacts as they fear inviting friends home or others finding out; and anger and frustration, may also be part of the younger person's experience. The effects on younger family members may not be immediately apparent but may be manifested in more subtle behaviour changes, such as decline in school performance, complaint of physical symptoms or withdrawal from family relationships.

The approach to supporting children and adolescents lies in communicating. Providing an explanation in language that the younger person can understand will enable their appreciation of changes to the family routine and the older persons' behaviour; technical and medical terminology are unlikely to be helpful. Many of the organisations under the umbrella of Alzheimer's Disease International (http://www.alz.co.uk/) provide information sheets directly aimed at younger people who live with the effects of dementia. Such information focuses on giving a brief explanation of the disease as affecting the brain and causing difficulties for the person in remembering, talking or taking care of themselves and pointing out that the person may see or hear things that are not there. The younger person is likely to have questions about what is happening. Providing a reason for what is happening is important and allowing them time to discuss events means that their needs can be identified and taken into account.

It should be recognised that changes to the role of individual family members as a result of dementia may result in a change of role for the child. They may have to take on more responsibility for themselves or contribute more to completing tasks about the home. This could obviously have a negative impact on younger family members, but equally could contribute to a more positive relationship with the person with dementia, particularly where there is an opportunity for enjoying shared activity. Younger children are less likely to stigmatise the person with dementia and to accept behaviour that is different to the norm. For example, a young child learning to dress themselves can appreciate just how difficult it is to do up buttons or get clothes on in the right order. They know that crossing the road alone or finding the way to and from the shops is a challenge. While encountering an adult with these difficulties may be unusual, they will understand the complexities the adult faces. Indeed, they are perhaps best placed to calmly help the older person achieve these tasks. While other members of the family are busier than usual absorbing the role of caregiver, the oldest and youngest may have time to undertake activities together: listening to music, a craft project, a walk or undertaking household chores. Such activities provide important opportunities for those involved. The child spends time in pleasurable pursuits, enjoys the time and attention of the adult and can feel they are contributing to the family. The person with dementia can feel useful, can pass on aspects of their life history and utilise their abilities. For both there is the potential to raise self-esteem and to learn from one another.

Older children and adolescents can face unique difficulties when a family member develops dementia. Teenage years are traditionally a time of life when communicating is hard and the effects of stigma, of anything being different from your peer group, is extremely challenging. For most, getting through these years is traumatic enough without the added strain of dementia in the family. They may be expected to grow up quickly, reduce the time spent with friends or on school work and take on extra responsibility. The emotions generated may include anger, sadness, embarrassment and guilt. Again within the research there is little to guide approaches aimed specifically at the needs of adolescents, but encouraging communication and reducing the risk of isolation from either the family or their peer group is likely to be important.

Evidence for Practice

The Younger Person's Experience of Dementia

Children and adolescents experience dementia when parents, grandparents or significant other family members have dementia

Dementia impacts on the child's relationship not only with the person with dementia but with others within the family

Children may feel angry, frightened, jealous, sad, frustrated, guilty or embarrassed

Emotions may not be directly expressed but changes in behaviour, school performance and physical health complaints may be apparent

Younger family members may have to take on more responsibility, for themselves or in caring for others

Children and adolescents need information about dementia, but the information should be appropriate to the age of the child

CONCLUSION

By recognising that people at all stages of dementia have an awareness of what is happening to them and that they retain a sense of self, we are learning to work in partnership with persons with dementia. By acknowledging the experience of individuals, we are learning to offer appropriate support to enable them to maintain an optimum quality of life and to live as positively as possible with dementia. We are learning not only what we have long suspected, that it is truly awful to be diagnosed with and to try to live with dementia, but also that the human being is truly remarkable in developing ways of coping with dementia and indeed enjoying aspects of living despite the potentially overwhelming experience of loss.

Research shows us that at different stages and different ages people living with dementia have differing needs. This enables care providers to target resources at meeting specific needs that are based on knowledge of the experience of dementia from the perspective of people who have dementia. This is a major advance and an important development in dementia care. No longer should services be developed based on the experience of those of us outside looking in or evaluated by those of us who provide but do not use the service.

Referring to people with dementia in terms of being a burden results in yet another negative label being added to a sector of society already carrying considerable stigma. Certainly being a caregiver for someone with dementia presents unique challenges, but concentrating research and intervention on the negative outcomes for carers ignores the positive experiences of caring and reduces the caring relationship to a one-dimensional condition in which the needs of the carer are paramount. There is a significant need to develop research into the dynamics of the caring relationship in the dementia specialism, not least because it seems likely that the focus of research questioning to date has been too narrow. It has concentrated on one element of the relationship, the carer, to the exclusion of others involved, primarily the cared for but also the needs and contributions of significant others, such as children and grandchildren. In closing it can be surmised that while we have come a long way we certainly have a long way yet to go before the experience of the person with dementia is fully influential in care practice and development.

6 Issues in Communication

INTRODUCTION

The learning curve for those working with people with dementia has been steep over the past 10 years. Research into the psychosocial dimensions of life with dementia has challenged those developing and providing care to do so in new and very different ways. Long held beliefs about what it is like to live with dementia have been turned on their head. As carers we must acknowledge that some of our past behaviour was based on ill-founded beliefs and has had a detrimental effect on those in our care. We must also acknowledge that in the face of what we now know there is pressure to change our behaviour and change quickly.

One aspect of our behaviour in need of urgent change is the way in which we communicate and establish relationships with people who have dementia. This chapter discusses the impact of dementia on communication and the barriers that exist as a result of this impact. These barriers come from areas that include the impact of dementia on the person with dementia, the impact of dementia on carers' perceptions and expectations of individuals with dementia and the barriers created by the manner in which organisations prioritise and deliver care services. These barriers are for once not easily overcome by employing research-based practice, primarily because the range of research currently available is not specific enough to give practitioners clear guidelines and strategies to overcome the barriers. The lack of support from the evidence base has not deterred practitioners from pursuing several approaches to aid their communication with people with dementia, including reminiscence therapy, validation therapy, music therapy, memory book work and psychotherapy. These approaches are also considered in this chapter.

The term 'challenging behaviour' has become common in the language of the dementia care specialism and the management of such behaviour has been a key role of caring services, particularly institutional and specialist mental health care services. The most common method of managing this behaviour has traditionally been through the use of tranquillising medication. However, a new interpretation of challenging behaviour is leading to a fresh understanding of such behaviour as a communication attempt. This chapter also considers this and the growing recognition that responding to this behaviour as a communication attempt requires new skills from carers. The chapter begins by examining the importance of communication in relation to care of individuals with dementia.

THE IMPORTANCE OF COMMUNICATION

We saw in Chapter 5 that it is important to develop ways of communicating effectively with people who have dementia, because to do so supports our ability to work in partnership in progressing services and evaluating their effectiveness. The evidence offers us, arguably, more important reasons for developing such communication. Communication is the foundation of social relationships; it is by communicating with others that we seek and secure social contact and it is through social contact and socially inclusive relationships that our place and value in the world is confirmed. Lack of meaningful social relationships threatens the individual's sense of self. Unless people with dementia are offered the opportunity and support to communicate and sustain social contact their very identity is threatened, self-esteem cannot be maintained and their quality of life is seriously endangered. As Ward *et al.* (2002) identify:

> Without meaningful communication, effectively we lose our place in the social world. From this perspective, the responsibilities involved in caring for someone with dementia are far deeper and wider than the task of providing 'care'. Poor communication, or a lack of interaction, carries serious ethical implications.

Sabat (2002) supports this view, describing how the various social personae we construct in the variety of situations in which we live our lives are dependent on the cooperation of others in our social world. For example, I could not maintain a sense of myself as a 'knowledgeable nurse' if at least some of my patients did not recognise me as a nurse or, as Sabat exemplifies, you could not construct the self of 'dedicated teacher' if one's students did not recognise you as being their teacher. The relevance of this in our communication with people with dementia is that if we view individuals with dementia as burdensome, challenging or somehow less of a person because of their having dementia, then their ability to hold on to their sense of who they are in the social world is seriously threatened and potentially lost. It is clear that this happens not because of the process of dementia but because those around the person with dementia cease communicating with them as the individual that they have always been, cease reinforcing the positive contributions the person makes to their social environment or indeed cease to give the individual the opportunity to make a contribution. Under these circumstances the individual is left with a sense of themselves purely as someone with dementia, damaged, burdensome and insignificant.

Kitwood (1997) reflected this when he defined 'personhood' as 'a standing or status that is bestowed upon one human being, by others, in the context of relationship and social being'. As those inhabiting the social world of an individual with dementia it is vital that we recognise that we are directly responsible for their place in that world, for it is through our behaviour, the quality and quantity of communication and social contact we offer that the individual will receive confirmation or otherwise of their value as a human being.

A further factor for consideration is the importance of communication in the relationship between the person with dementia and their carer, particularly where care is undertaken in the home. There is evidence that a breakdown in communication leads to the carer surrendering the caring role. Where communication breaks down and the carer is unable to establish meaningful communication their ability to recognise the individual that they know and love is threatened. This threat has been shown to lead to the carer surrendering the caring role, potentially sooner than would have been the case if communication had been sustained.

Before we move on it is important that we acknowledge a final possible consequence of not providing an opportunity for communication and social inclusion for people with dementia. The nature of dementia is that it is progressive; the longer you live with dementia the greater the disability you suffer is likely to be. As we considered in Chapter 3, there has been a growing consensus over the past few years that such an explanation is too simple in terms of describing exactly how dementia affects individuals. Investigations carried out post-mortem have found that severe damage to the brain does not necessarily equate to severe symptoms of dementia; this points to factors other than brain damage by dementia being responsible for exacerbating symptoms. Studies into the psychosocial factors impacting on people who have dementia indicate that poor social relationships and exclusion exacerbate the effects of dementia. Accepting this should make us consider the importance of sustaining communication, supporting individuality and enabling individuals with dementia to remain in contact with the world around them.

Evidence for Practice

The Importance of Communication

Effective communication with people who have dementia enables services to be developed and evaluated in partnership

Communication is vital in keeping individuals in touch with the social world and in confirming their place in it

Effective communication sustains individuality and validates a sense of self

Breakdown in communication can result in family carers resorting to institutional care

We, as the people who form the individual's contact with the social world, are directly responsible for their inclusion in that world and confirming that they are valued human beings

Breakdown in communication can result in an exacerbation of symptoms of dementia

---

THE IMPACT OF DEMENTIA ON THE INDIVIDUAL'S COMMUNICATION ABILITY

Dementia impacts on communication in many ways, the most obvious being that the damage to the brain that dementia brings means that an individual's ability to use and interpret verbal and nonverbal language is progressively eroded. The manner in which memory is disrupted by dementia influences the individual's ability to communicate successfully. Semantic memory, the system through which our knowledge of the world is stored, is impaired by dementia. For people with dementia this means knowledge of the meaning of words and the rules and concepts that enable them to construct a mental representation of the world in an abstract way is damaged. This can result in difficulty with both spoken and written communication, leading to language seeming vague and the use of few words or words that are difficult to understand. As dementia progresses, initiating and sustaining conversation becomes hard and sticking to the subject difficult. The volume of verbal output is reduced and ideas and words may become repetitive. The temptation is to regard such communication as unimportant or meaningless.

Episodic memory, the part of memory that stores autobiographical details and lets us remember events that were personally experienced at a specific time and place, is also adversely affected by dementia. While specific events from long ago may be remembered, increasingly more and more support from others is required to sustain even these memories.

Much is made of the loss of short term memory in dementia, but how it actually impacts on communication has implications for how we give information. For example, using sentences that give several pieces of information at once demands an ability to understand the words (semantic memory) and also the ability to retain the sentence long enough to extract the different pieces of information, make sense of them and formulate an appropriate response. Given a difficulty with retaining in the short term this can be almost impossible as dementia progresses.

Memory is an extremely complex function and depends on many parts of the brain to operate effectively. When memory function begins to be damaged by dementia the impact on the individual's life and particularly on communication ability is significant. Memory is not the only factor impacting on the success of communication. A decline in attention span and the capacity to concentrate affects the manner in which information is absorbed and the person's ability to follow the thread of a conversation or social activity; thus the individual's participation in social communication is compromised.

The shrinking of the individual's social world compounded by the stigma that is attached to having dementia reduces the opportunities that most people with dementia have to be involved in conversation and to be included socially. An individual's initial response to having dementia is often to withdraw from social situations. Individuals with dementia are likely to be reluctant to keep putting themselves in situations where they repeatedly experience difficulty understanding others and getting others to understand them, where their control of language and memory frequently fails them. Equally other people are likely to be embarrassed by the communication difficulties of the person who has dementia and, not knowing how to respond, may seek to avoid them.

We must also consider the potential impact of other age related changes, particularly where the person with dementia is over 65, for example hearing and sight changes. In a 1995 study Gates *et al.* found that in common with older adults in the general population 30 % of people with dementia aged between 65 and 74 years have hearing loss and that percentage rises to more than 50 % in those aged more than 75 years. On a more worrying note Hopper *et al.* (2001) found that people with dementia who had hearing and speech difficulties in nursing homes were not referred for specialist treatment. If this study proves representative of the nature of attention paid to such basic needs and disregard for the importance of seeking specialist services for people with dementia then there is indeed cause for concern, particularly as Gates *et al.* observe, because hearing and cognition are so closely related that deficiencies in one area can affect performance in the other.

We have considered previously in this book the impact and frequency of depression in dementia and in considering an individual's communication needs we should bear in mind that where depression is present communication will be negatively affected. We have also considered that lack of social opportunity leads to depression in people with dementia and that provision of suitable social activity may be more important in treating this cause of depression than other methods. If we are not careful this problem becomes self-perpetuating; people with dementia develop depression because of lack of opportunity and support in meaningful social communication and depression leads to a reduced ability of the individual to participate in social communication.

The barriers dementia enforces on individuals with respect to limiting communication are most frequently associated with deterioration in speech, comprehension and memory ability. For the individual this means they have fewer words at their disposal and great difficulty constructing and interpreting sentences. As we saw in the opening chapter, stigma associated with mental illness and old age already disadvantages those with dementia; communication difficulties add to stigma and further marginalise people who have dementia. The implications of this difficulty with communicating for the individual are significant from the perspective of achieving social contact and inclusion and it is not hard to conclude that people with dementia are unlikely to be able to overcome these barriers alone.

Evidence for Practice

The Impact of Dementia on Communication

Dementia related changes to memory cause difficulty in the use of verbal and written language

Loss of short term memory causes the individual difficulty in interpreting sentences that involve more than one piece of information or instruction

As dementia progresses fewer words are used and conversation may be vague and repetitive

Changes in the ability to concentrate may result in difficulty sustaining conversation or sticking to the subject

Memory for autobiographical events is progressively impaired as a result of dementia

Shrinking of the individual's social circle together with dementia related stigma reduces opportunities for communication and social inclusion

People with dementia may not have access to specialist help with hearing and sight loss

Depression can be caused by social exclusion and impairs the ability to communicate

ORGANISATIONAL BARRIERS TO COMMUNICATION

Barriers to communication come not only as a consequence of dementia but as a consequence of our perceptions and expectations of people who have dementia. We as carers, particularly carers in institutional settings, create and maintain as many barriers to communication and social inclusion as the dementia itself. As has already been seen, the research identifying that persons with dementia retain a sense of self is relatively recent and has still not infiltrated all care practice. It is still widely believed that people with dementia do not function as 'normal' human beings who have an appreciation and opinion of what is happening to and around them. The behaviour and communication attempts of people with dementia are recognised as symptomatic of the disease rather than valid efforts at making contact and sustaining relationships with others. Continuing to harbour such impressions about people with dementia precludes our appreciation of the need or possibility of involving them in social communication and including them in social activity.

The manner in which we organise care settings, with high priority being given to achieving tasks aimed at meeting basic needs for nutrition, safety and hygiene, creates huge obstacles for communication. Institutional care settings are structured, almost exclusively, towards meeting these needs. Levels of staffing, types of furniture, environmental layout, visiting arrangements, mealtimes – the list is endless as everything is focused towards meeting physical needs. The structure of the environments we expect people with dementia to live in when they can no longer live at home do not lend themselves to supporting social communication, let alone provide that extra level of assistance that people with dementia require to sustain meaningful contact with others. Consider, for example, the use of a television or radio in institutional settings, where the volume frequently prevents individuals from striking up a conversation. Consider seating arrangements, often suited to accomplishing care tasks and allowing carers' easy access between clients' chairs, but which mean that individuals cannot have eye contact with others with whom they might converse or where the person nearest to them is still too far away to make conversation possible. We know that in institutional care settings mealtimes are an occasion that can prompt communication between patients, but we need to acknowledge that apart from the social aspect of mealtimes the mere fact that individuals are seated close to each other and can see and hear each other are vital to supporting communication.

Indeed, much of the communication that does take place between the carer and the person with dementia is centred on tending to physical care needs. Morse and Intrieri (1997) reported that on average the time spent in a nurse–patient interaction in long term care facilities was less than 30 minutes per day. Ward *et al.* (2005) found that the most consistent contact people with dementia had was with care workers and that this communication accounted for approximately 2 % of the day. More worryingly, 78 % of this communication was centred on achieving a care task. Furthermore, where the person with dementia was familiar with the routine of the task even less communication was offered as the carer could complete the task without having to instruct the person in what to do, meaning that up to two-thirds of the communication that did take place was nonverbal. Interestingly, Ward *et al.* also found that poor understanding or failure on the part of the person with dementia to comply in getting the task done led to increased communication aimed at achieving the task. It could therefore be construed that people with dementia have something to gain by refusing to cooperate with care staff, because to do so results in an increased opportunity for communication, even if some of that communication is aimed at getting the person to do something they do not want to do.

While the Ward *et al.* study revealed some examples of interaction that were posi-tive, warm and tender, such examples were infrequent and led them to conclude that: 'Relationships between care staff and people with dementia residing in care were shaped almost entirely by what seemed to us the "mantra" of dementia care: *out of bed – wash – dress – feed – toilet – back to bed.*' This study is not an isolated account confirming the level and nature of communication between care staff and people with dementia in 24-hour care settings, but given that it is recent and against a background of the overwhelming body of new information available for carers in these settings it is shocking. What is clear is that, particularly in 24-hour care settings, people with dementia spend only a fraction of their day in communication with others. Those others are primarily care staff and the communication that does take place is largely concerned with enabling care staff to accomplish a specific physical care task.

A further barrier to communication with people with dementia is the context within which we, as potential communication partners, place the issue. If we believe that the problem lies in the inability of the person with dementia then we are more likely to subscribe to the 'no cure no hope' school of thought and assume little can be done. However, if we accept that the difficulties lie not in the individual's inability to communicate but in our inability to interpret communication that is influenced by dementia, and if we acknowledge that our contribution, particularly in 24-hour care settings, is inadequate then a shift in approach becomes necessary.

The evidence leaves us in little doubt that people with dementia continue to attempt communication using whatever means remain available to them. If communication is not achieved it is because those of us who do not have dementia are not making sufficient effort to get past the restrictions imposed by the individual's dementia to find the method of communication that will enable contact to be made. We are beginning to understand that the aim of communication with people with dementia should be to involve them in social activity that promotes their feelings of self-worth, that sustains their individuality, that enables them to retain a sense of their value in their social group and that ultimately sustains good life quality. An examination of the evidence reveals several significant barriers to meaningful communication with people who have dementia; the barriers dementia brings, the mental barriers carers carry in relation to expectations of people with dementia and the barriers that a persistence in prioritising care in task-based activity enforces all lead to poor understanding and appreciation of the need to create opportunities for communication. What is very clear is that the person who has dementia bears no responsibility for the persistence of these barriers; it is certainly not their fault that they have dementia. What is clear is that as carers it is we who have responsibility for overcoming and dismantling these barriers. To do so we are required to develop skills specific to interpreting communication that is disrupted by dementia and to reorganise and reprioritise care tasks to highlight the importance of creating an opportunity to communicate in order to develop and use our understanding of the importance of social inclusion for people with dementia. As far back as 1969 Ruddock identified that man has two social needs that are so important that they are rated higher than the need to survive, these being the need to feel that existence is of some significance and the need to have enduring relationships. It could be construed that while we are very busy ensuring the physical survival of those in our care who have dementia we are doing little to provide enduring relationships or relationships within which the person with dementia can feel that their existence is of any significance.

Evidence for Practice

Organisational Barriers to Communication

The perceptions and expectations carers have of people with dementia can create barriers to effective communication

As carers we continue to consider the communication attempts of people with dementia as symptomatic of their disease rather than valid attempts to interact, despite evidence to the contrary

The organisation and prioritising of carers' time and energy around physical care tasks are instrumental in creating and sustaining barriers to effective communication

Repeated studies into the level and nature of communication in institutional care settings show that in fact it is task orientated and as little as 2 % of a care recipient's day is spent on communicating – this should shock us

People who have dementia are not responsible for a breakdown in communication

We, as carers, are responsible for a breakdown in communication and we have not only the power to overcome and dismantle the barriers but an ethical obligation to do so

DIFFICULTIES WITH THE RESEARCH

Research contributes to the progression of care practice by seeking to answer questions about care situations, approaches to care and the outcomes for recipients and providers of care. In this way research provides clinicians with information that enables decisions to be made about situations and approaches and whether they are achieving desired outcomes. In simple terms research helps us to recognise when situations and approaches need to be changed, because what is happening is not achieving a positive outcome for those involved in the care relationship. We can see an example of this process in the way change is occurring in the area of diagnosis disclosure. Once research began to ask questions about the pros and cons of disclosure clinicians began to respond to the information research provided and to change practice towards disclosure rather than continue with the accepted practice of nondisclosure. Research is a powerful tool in pinpointing a need to change and in directing clinicians in the best method of achieving the required change. However, the research into communication with people with dementia is largely fragmented and often contradictory, which is leading to difficulty for clinicians in taking information and applying it to practice.

Most textbooks and training programmes specific to health and social care, targeted at registered and unregistered staff, include information on the skills required to communicate with older adults. Attention is drawn to the ways in which trainees can use verbal and nonverbal behaviour to establish relationships that will facilitate the delivery of the care or treatment needed by the client.

The factors considered important include verbal content and how it is delivered, means of conveying information nonverbally to support verbal expression and to reflect interest in and empathy with the other person, methods of attracting the other person's attention and keen listening skills to aid interpretation of the communication of others. Touch is considered important but a measured approach is recommended as being key to its use, and there is advice on how to limit the impact of environmental disturbances and how to use elements within the environment (for example positioning chairs) to promote better communication. These techniques have long been presented as the skills required by clinicians to enhance their communication with people with mental health problems, people with dementia included. For the majority of clinicians working in other areas of mental health these skills form the basic toolkit upon which to build effective communication. Counselling skills and more intensive, expert psychotherapeutic and cognitive interventions were added and employed, with clients depending on the need and level of expertise of the practitioner. However, in the world of dementia care, traditionally no benefit was seen in developing more expert methods of communication. Although there is now some evidence of change and some examples of methods of enhancing communication with people with dementia, the basic toolkit is the one that the majority of carers have at their disposal on a daily basis.

Whether employing these skills actually produces the desired outcomes in creating and sustaining the type of support people with dementia need with regard to overcoming barriers to communicating is open to debate, particularly as there is little evidence from research that supports the use of such skills. It is unclear why there should be such a lack of evidence, apart from the fact that most of the skills demanded amount to the basic tenets of reasonable communication and so there seems to be a universal, unproven agreement that they constitute the correct method of approach. It seems there is significant evidence to support the view that we do not communicate effectively with people with dementia, not least because it has taken us so long to uncover some very important information about the experience of dementia and in many areas spend only a tiny proportion of our day actually involved in communication with people with dementia.

A major criticism of research studies into aspects of dementia care, in particular studies that seek information about communication-based psychosocial interventions, is that they infrequently meet the criteria for randomised controlled trials and are undertaken with too few study subjects to be meaningful in the wider context. Warner *et al.* (2005) also express concern that people involved in research into treatments for dementia are not representative of the population of people with dementia. They point out that few randomised controlled trials are undertaken in primary care and that the majority are conducted with people with Alzheimer's disease rather than other types of dementia.

As a result many of the accepted psychosocial interventions commonly used in dementia care are not evidence based, including reality orientation, reminiscence therapy and music therapy. As an example consider the review undertaken by Vink *et al.* (2003) of music therapy for people with dementia. They concluded that: 'The methodological quality and the reporting of the included studies were too poor to draw any useful conclusions.' The difficulty therefore lies not just in ensuring that we use research to ask the correct question, which is undoubtedly vital, but also that we undertake research using methodology that can unequivocally deliver answers that can be applied to our practice.

The difficulty of where to seek support in developing strategies for communicating with people with dementia that do work is also compounded by pieces of work that seem to offer contradictory advice. For example, Sheldon (1994) found that transmitting complex thoughts and directions by simple phrases was effective but Perry *et al.* (2005) found that it was possible to communicate effectively using complex grammatical structures. Similarly, studies into the value of using yes–no questions as opposed to open-ended questions yield apparently contradictory results. However, the findings of Allan (2001) may shed light on these apparently contradictory results. In exploring ways carers could consult with persons with dementia Allan found that the response to communication approaches using both verbal and nonverbal forms varied at different times and in different circumstances. Allan also noted that it was important to know the individual's strengths and needs with regard to communication, that the individual's interests and background required consideration and that the nature of the person's relationship with the carer impacted on the success of the communication.

Strategies that include providing an opportunity for the person to communicate, listening to what is said, attending to the context within which it is said and accepting that behaviour, no matter how bizarre, as an effort to say something offer the way forward. To such strategies must be added a knowledge of the individual's past experiences. Allan also identified that it is necessary to address organisational barriers and to support staff in using the opportunities that do present themselves.

What may be of significance also is that researchers are now beginning to ask whether the manner in which questions are posed or information is given can influence the success of communication. One such study by Small and Perry (2005) set out to examine whether the demands made on the individual's memory would influence the choice of strategy chosen to communicate. Thus one of the hypotheses Small and Perry set out to test was whether a more positive communication outcome would occur when carers used questions that requested information from *semantic* memory rather than *episodic* memory. The results showed that the use of questions demanding a response from semantic memory, that part of memory that stores general world knowledge, were more effective in sustaining conversation than questions demanding a response involving episodic memory, that part of memory storing information linked to a specific time, place, person or event in the past. They established that open-ended questions (previously advised against) that relied on a response from semantic memory were more successful than yes–no questions (previously encouraged as supporting communication) that relied on episodic memory.

This is important as it leads us to examine the nature of memory more closely and to see how it interrupts communication and leads us to working with the person's retained ability. It would also explain why similar studies are throwing up apparently contradictory information. It is not necessarily the manner in which the question is posed (open-ended or requiring a yes–no answer) but the subject matter of the questions and the individual's potential for using retained memory ability to respond to the subject matter that is important.

Once we begin to appreciate what happens to people's abilities to communicate as a result of dementia we can begin to use this knowledge to improve the way we communicate, in particular in working to identify how communication can be sustained by working with retained strengths and in working to compensate for loss of ability. While research obviously benefits effective care practice, in turn it is led by clinicians seeking answers to specific questions. In respect of communication we have achieved answers to several questions. Can people with dementia communicate at all stages of dementia? Yes they can. Is communication important in maintaining esteem and self-worth? Yes it is. Do we support the communication needs of people with dementia, particularly in 24-hour care settings? No we do not. Clinicians need to generate a fuller list of questions that could be addressed by research studies in order to inform practice around communication fully. This will lead to an enriched evidence base of strategies, principles and guidelines from which to compile approaches to care.

In many ways it is easy to be critical of the paucity of information the evidence base offers for those of us seeking to improve our communication skills. We should remember, however, that the importance of communication and sustaining social contact with people who have dementia is still in the process of being fully understood. Our previous understanding of the communication needs of people with dementia has been that we need to communicate to accomplish physical care tasks. This is very different from what is likely to be required if we want to sustain social contact, sustain personhood and confirm the value of individuals. Communication that supports and nourishes holistically is very different from communication that nourishes the body, and many diverse factors require consideration.

Information that can enlighten communication techniques must therefore address factors related to the individual, including personality, abilities and needs, circumstances, life history, past and current relationships, potential new relationships and the opportunities that exist or can be created to facilitate communication. Research into activity for people with dementia also has much to offer those seeking successful communication with people with dementia. The expertise, knowledge and training of carers and research into their needs and factors impacting on success of communication must also be reflected upon. Giving these factors consideration within an evidence seeking format will take time.

TECHNIQUES COMMONLY USED IN DEMENTIA CARE

While we may be critical of the overall range and quality of information provided thus far by the research base to help us overcome the barriers to communication that dementia brings, we can certainly find examples of instances where practitioners have investigated specific techniques and found them beneficial, even if this benefit is unproven from the scientific perspective. These examples demonstrate that clinicians have an interest in and are motivated to seek interventions that support their communication with people with dementia but lack specialist skills in delivering results in a form that will enable them to be credible and transferable. It should also be acknowledged that while there is little support for the efficacy of these techniques within the evidence base this does not automatically mean that these techniques are ineffective. Some of the more popular techniques are presented below.

MEMORY BOOKS

It has been stressed throughout this and the preceding chapter that sustaining the individual's sense of themselves and their place in the social world is important. As we begin to understand that episodic memory is seriously threatened by dementia and indeed that the extent to which this threat impacts adversely on effective communication is great, we can begin to appreciate the need to find ways of prompting the use of episodic memory in order to sustain the individual's sense of who they are and to promote continued communication.

One technique that has a growing evidence base is the work of Michelle Bourgeois. A synopsis of the work of Bourgeois (2003) with referenced evidence provides some support for its effectiveness in sustaining communication with people with dementia and improving the quality of life. Bourgeois found that by use of a 'memory book' individual's difficulties with semantic memory and communication could be overcome.

The 'memory book' comprises a collection of pages, each with short written sentences and related photographs, that are presented in conversation to people with dementia. The words and photographs are highly personal and the language used simple and short. Bourgeois found that the individuals could read and relate to the pages, add detail and express thoughts they wanted to share. Carers using the memory books reported a positive effect on reducing levels of anxiety and agitation and decreasing the frequency of repeated questions on the part of the person with dementia. As an aid to communication Bourgeois concludes that her studies suggest 'that written input can access semantic information that is not accessible by other input modalities (i.e. auditory or verbal input) and can contribute to a better quality of life for persons with dementia and their caregivers'.

MUSIC THERAPY

Loiselle and Dupuis (2003) provide a synopsis of the importance of music as a communication tool with people with dementia. They identify music as a trigger for emotions and memories of people, places and events throughout an individual's lifetime. The power of music when viewed thus enables our understanding of its use as a means of communicating with people who as a result of dementia have difficulty evoking these memories voluntarily or using them in conversation to support their identity. Music therapy aims to produce positive outcomes for people with dementia in respect of their social and behavioural symptoms by compensating for the limitations dementia places on an individual's ability to act and express themselves. Loiselle and Dupuis cite evidence for music and music therapy as a method of enhancing language skills and improved ability to communicate, prompting an increase in talking, smiling, gesturing and other social skills that support communication. The use of music in dementia care varies from playing an individual's favourite music to sing-alongs, attendance at a concert or direct involvement in making music. In a review of the evidence for the effectiveness of nondrug therapies for dementia, Gräsel *et al.* (2003) found that a lack of controlled studies led to an inability to assess the effectiveness of music therapy in dementia care reliably.

VALIDATION THERAPY

We saw in Chapter 1 that validation therapy (VT) was one of the first attempts to establish communication with people who have dementia that addressed the needs of the individual. Despite being applied to practice over a period of some 30 years there is still little research evidence to support the application of VT in dementia care. Again, as Day (1997) identifies, this is largely as a result of poorly constructed research studies rather than an indictment of VT.

Naomi Feil, a gerontological social worker, developed the theory and techniques of VT, which was initially developed as an alternative to reality orientation. Reality orientation was seen as an attempt to bring individuals who suffer disorientation back to the present by repeatedly reminding them where they are, what is happening around them and the current date and time. VT suggests that this is not helpful for many old people and that, as an alternative, carers and clinicians should seek to enter the reality of the disorientated individual and support the emotions they are expressing and enable them to resolve painful emotions.

VT is presented as a theory on ageing, particularly old old age where progressive disorientation is a feature. An accompanying set of communication techniques are proposed to enable the individual to resolve life issues prior to death. Feil (1993) describes four stages of very old age: malorientation, time confusion, repetitive motion and vegetation. Validation techniques are underpinned by principles that include recognition that each person is unique and should be treated as an individual and each individual is valuable and there is reason behind all behaviour and each stage of life has particular psychological tasks that must be completed as failure to do so leads to psychological problems. For very old people the task is to resolve life issues. Validation theory suggests that in very old age where memory fails the individual restores balance and attempts to resolve life issues by retrieving past memories and that where these memories are expressed as painful they should be acknowledged and validated as this will diminish the pain. Furthermore, empathy is key to building trust which will reduce an individual's anxiety and restore dignity.

The benefits of validation therapy are described as improved verbal and nonverbal communication skills, reduced episodes of challenging behaviour such as crying, pacing and aggression, enabling individuals to resolve life tasks, reduction in an individual's levels of anxiety, an improved sense of self-worth, slowing down of the rate of deterioration and a reduced need to rely on restraint and psychotropic medication as methods of treatment. Benefits to staff employing validation techniques include improved morale and reduced burn-out.

Gräsel et al. (2003) reflect the view that 'the communicative aspect of the validation principle, based on empathy and unconditional esteem, is a plausible concept for dealing with dementia patients', but there are doubts about Feil's underpinning theory and assertions that using the techniques enables individuals with dementia to reconstruct past methods of coping to help them overcome present crises. As with many of the psychosocial approaches in dementia care we remain in need of empirical evidence that can be supplied only from a rigorous research base.

REMINISCENCE THERAPY

Reminiscence therapy has a rich background in the care of older adults, not only in dementia care but also in the care of older adults suffering from depression. In the treatment of depression reminiscence therapy is used primarily to encourage a life review, through which the individual can evaluate and analyse memories and with the aid of a therapist achieve a sense of integrity.

However, in dementia care the benefits of reminiscence are found in its application as a communication aid. It is proposed that talking about the past and re-living life events can support the individual's self-esteem and identity and enable an individual with dementia to utilise retained memory ability. Brooker (2001) identifies reminiscence as being distinct from life review in that reminiscence 'is seen as having a variety of goals, including increased communication and socialisation, and providing pleasure and entertainment'.

Techniques to stimulate reminiscence include asking open-ended questions, for example 'do you remember your first day at school?', or concentrating on historical events group members may have lived through, like the War years, the death of J.F. Kennedy or important local events. Memorabilia such as pictures, objects and newspapers can be introduced to group members to stimulate memories. Many commentators caution that involving individuals in reminiscence work should be balanced against what we know about the individual and care should be taken not to stimulate painful memories and emotions. However, painful memories and emotions will be expressed at times and the important element is not necessarily to avoid these situations but to provide the individual with emotional support and comfort when distress is expressed. In assessing the evidence for the effectiveness of reminiscence commentators can only call for more studies employing rigorous techniques to be undertaken. Again it is important to remember that inability to prove clinical effectiveness is not proof of ineffectiveness.

PSYCHOTHERAPY

Practising psychotherapy with people over the age of 65 is a relatively new phenomenon. Until 15 years ago psychotherapy with people with dementia was at best considered foolhardy. As a minimum psychotherapy requires the ability to remember and reflect upon matters discussed during therapy – abilities people with dementia are not capable of, or are they? In just 15 years we have come a long way, so far in fact that dementia now warrants a full chapter in recent books on psychotherapy for older adults (Garner, 2004).

The main drive in psychotherapeutic work with people with dementia has been in providing an emotionally safe place wherein the trauma of receiving a diagnosis of dementia can be absorbed. The work of Yale (1995) in the United States and Jones *et al.* (2002) in the United Kingdom have shown that groupwork based on psychotherapeutic principles is not only possible but effective in providing a place for individuals newly diagnosed with dementia to meet others in a similar situation, to express feelings and to share experiences. Jones *et al.* (2002) found evidence that as a result of participating in the support groups levels of anxiety and depression fell in group participants. The feedback from group participants provided in the form of comments by both Yale and Jones *et al.* speak volumes for the need and benefit of support groups for individuals with early dementia.

What we can conclude from consideration of these techniques developed specifically to support the communication needs of people who have dementia is that this is an area requiring both more investigation and corroboration. We certainly need to extend the skills of carers in establishing and sustaining communication and we definitely need to be sure that the processes we are using are effective. We should remember that while the research does not prove the effectiveness of these techniques or tell us which method is the best there is nothing in the research to say they are detrimental. As techniques that require we make contact and interact with persons who have dementia the use of reminiscence, music, validation and psychotherapeutic techniques should be encouraged as indispensable to our practice.

Evidence for Practice

Difficulties with Research

Research is a powerful tool in pinpointing a need to change and in directing clinicians in the best method of achieving the required change

People working in dementia care rely on a basic communication toolkit which is not confirmed by an evidence base

Research into communication with people with dementia is largely fragmented and often contradictory, making it difficult for practitioners to apply findings to their practice

Some pieces of research are beginning to shed light on the factors thought important when communicating with people who have dementia

Factors requiring consideration in relation to individuals with dementia are likely to include personality, abilities and needs, circumstances, life history and past, current and potential new relationships

Other factors requiring consideration include the opportunities that exist and can be created for communication and social activity to take place

The onus is on practitioners to generate the type of questions research can concentrate on to inform practice

The research evidence on the use of reminiscence therapy, music therapy, validation therapy and psychotherapeutic techniques in dementia care is inconclusive; these techniques should be used on the basis that they require exponents to communicate with people who have dementia

---

CHALLENGING BEHAVIOUR OR COMMUNICATION?

Challenging behaviour is the term used to describe activity on the part of persons with dementia that increases the burden of care. From the carer's perspective the challenge is to address and stop such activity so that the task of undertaking care becomes more manageable and the stress associated with the burden of care is reduced. It is also considered beneficial to the person with dementia that this activity is controlled and they no longer need to behave in such negative ways.

The traditional explanation for behaviour termed 'challenging' is that it occurs as a result of the damage caused to the brain by dementia; it is symptomatic of dementia syndrome. As we have seen, practice built on *traditional* explanations of what happens to people as a result of dementia is increasingly being brought into question. Several types of behaviour are considered challenging. These include aggression, wandering, shouting, repetitive verbalisation or questioning, repetitive actions, disturbed sleeping, food refusal, inappropriate sexual behaviour and incontinence. Within each of these categories of behaviour there are descriptive characteristics. Aggression includes verbal and physical violence, swearing, hitting, slapping, punching, being resistive, biting and scratching, for example. Wandering is used to describe individuals who attempt to walk for long periods of the day and night, often regardless of the fact that they cannot do so safely. This category of behaviour is also used to describe individuals who constantly seek to exit their current environment. Shouting behaviour includes shouting for prolonged periods of time for no apparent reason and often with no apparent external stimulus. Repetitive questioning, repeating apparently empty phrases or undertaking actions again and again that bear no relation to the individual's environment or the current context of their lives is considered challenging. A poor sleep pattern, particularly night time waking, is considered a challenging behaviour. Food refusal, eating inappropriate items and other undesirable food related behaviour, such as cramming food into the mouth, spitting food out or making a mess while eating, is deemed problematic for carers and is thus labelled as challenging. Incontinence and behaviour that occurs around toilet needs, such as spreading faeces or urinating in inappropriate places, are deemed to create so many challenges for carers that care at home frequently ceases to be an option once such behaviour is manifest. Even facilities designed specifically for people with dementia, such as day centres and residential homes, frequently refuse to offer places to individuals with this behaviour. Behaving in a sexually inappropriate manner, for example making comments with sexual connotations, touching staff inappropriately or touching or displaying genitalia, is termed challenging. There are numerous outcomes for people with dementia who behave in these ways, not least that they themselves become labelled as 'challenging'. For many family carers the manifestation of challenging behaviour is the point at which they feel forced to opt for institutional care.

If we are not going to accept the traditional premise of approaches to challenging behaviour that explain this behaviour in terms of a result of damage that dementia causes the brain, how else might we construct an explanation for this behaviour? The research offers us a clear alternative and that is that such behaviour is a means of communicating the experience of the individual with regard to what is happening to them and an attempt to express needs.

In discussing what he called the old culture of dementia care, Kitwood (1995) proposed that approaches were designed to control problem behaviour rather than to seek 'to understand the message, and so to engage with the need that is not being met'. The focus of attention should not therefore be the behaviour per se, rather carers must seek to uncover the need that is driving the behaviour and recognise that the behaviour is the means by which individuals with dementia continue to try and communicate their experience of what is happening to and around them and to express what they need when attempts at conventional communication are beyond their ability or are unsuccessfully interpreted by carers.

In many ways challenging behaviour as a communication tool is extremely effective in that it focuses our attention on the individual, but if we respond to challenging behaviour as a symptom of the dementing process we choose to ignore the underlying message the person is attempting to communicate. It is a growing realisation of this and recognition of this behaviour as a valid attempt to communicate that is demanding change in carers' responses to challenging behaviour. What is needed from us as carers is that we make efforts to decipher the need behind the behaviour, as meeting this need has the potential to resolve the challenging behaviour.

In pursuit of explanations for the more common challenging behaviours, Stokes (2000) investigates the possible meaning and need underlying the behaviour. He dissects the difficulties that dementia presents for the individual in getting specific needs met. It therefore becomes easier for us to understand that challenging behaviour is, in fact, a reasonable response by people who have dementia to the challenges that *they* face, not only as a result of having dementia but not infrequently as a result of the behaviour of carers.

As an example Stokes explores possible explanations for aggression and suggests that aggression may stem from multiple factors. It may be an attempt by the individual to defend themselves when their personal space is invaded and when, without explanation, others set about delivering care of an intimate nature (during a toileting activity for example) it may be a reaction to their own incompetence being highlighted or a response to others denying them the opportunity to complete an action they are intent upon. With regard to repetitive questioning, Stokes suggests this behaviour may stem from short term memory impairment, from boredom or from an attempt to engage with others and retain human contact. Similarly, constant walking may have its origin in anxiety prompted by loss of contact with familiar people or environment or may be a result of confusion where the individual seeks someone or something from their past. They may be driven by the need to collect children from school or find deceased loved ones as a result of this confusion; responding with orientation information in this instance can be considered harmful. However, by employing empathy we can begin to understand what is motivating the individual to be constantly on the go.

Viewed in this manner challenging behaviour is quite clearly related to the individual's difficulty with communication. An inability to control language and to make sense of the language of others necessitates the individual's reliance on other methods to communicate their needs and opinions. To exemplify, if I have dementia and I am unable to understand your communication that you intend to take me to the toilet, but you take me anyway and in so doing invade my personal space, interfere with my clothing and touch me in intimate places, if at the same time I do not agree that I need to go to the toilet and I do not have the use of language that will let us negotiate the meeting of this need to both our satisfaction, can you be surprised that I react to your actions, in an aggressive manner? In order to express my need to maintain my dignity, assert my wishes and to reject your actions, the only means available to me is aggression. Our developing knowledge of what it is like to live with dementia should tell us that this response was entirely predictable and that the fault lies with carers for not seeking to explore ways where the task could have been undertaken with a better outcome for both carer and cared for.

A final aspect of behaviour to consider, one not immediately perceived as challenging, is social withdrawal. Individuals with dementia, who withdraw completely from social interaction, even to the point of offering no objection to what happens to and around them, are not generally considered to be challenging individuals. There is little about their behaviour that increases the burden or the stress of caring and complete withdrawal from social communication does not inhibit the completion of tasks within a care environment. On the contrary, it may be seen as desirable as the individual offers no discernible objection to what happens to them. It must, however, be considered one of the most extreme responses of the person with dementia and we could interpret this withdrawal as the final relinquishing of the self to circumstance. This behaviour is characterised by lack of interest in the environment, cessation of the use of language, although occasional words let us know the person can articulate, and a response to the communication of others that reflects awareness of the other but makes no effort to reciprocate communication. This probably results from extended periods of time where the person did try to communicate socially but was ignored and events happened to and around the person that denied their agency, leaving them with the knowledge that they were totally unable to influence their own lives. This withdrawal does not command our attention in the care environment in the way that aggression or shouting does and it is easy to imagine that the person's quietness is a sign of contentment. It is not and should be interpreted as a sign that they have given up completely. This is certainly an aspect of the dementia care specialism requiring more research, both into the cause of the behaviour and how to care for the individuals exhibiting it.

Evidence for Practice

Challenging Behaviour

The term 'challenging' is used to label people who have dementia when the way in which they behave increases the burden and stress of care

Challenging behaviour includes aggression, constant walking, shouting, food refusal, sexually inappropriate behaviour, repetitive actions or questioning, disturbed sleep and incontinence

The traditional explanation for challenging behaviour is that it results as a consequence of dementia

Challenging behaviour is now recognised as a communication attempt

Carers must look beyond the behaviour to identify and respond to the underlying need the individual is communicating

Approaches to challenging behaviour must be individual

Social withdrawal is a form of challenging behaviour frequently overlooked

APPROACHES TO RESOLVING CHALLENGING BEHAVIOUR

The traditional treatment for challenging behaviours has been the use of medication aimed at pacifying the individual, making their behaviour more acceptable and enabling care tasks to be easily achieved. These drugs are largely antipsychotic preparations indicated for use in treating schizophrenia, bipolar disorder and psychoses in adults. For two primary reasons such a pharmaceutical approach is inappropriate. Firstly, this approach denies the underlying needs the individual is trying to communicate and can only control the behaviour, leaving the individual with unmet needs and with even less ability to express those needs as the effect of the medication compromises the individual's verbal, physical and emotional expression. Added to this is the fact that these drugs are not licensed for use in people with dementia. Secondly, the increasing information from pharmacological studies warns against the use of the drugs of choice as having poor outcomes on life expectancy for older adults. Bullock (2005) warns that trials reflect an increased likelihood of cerebrovascular adverse events.

Bird *et al.* (1998) suggest that the habitual recourse to psychotropic medication practised in most nursing home facilities for elderly patients is conditioned by an entrenched medical and nursing culture rather than any particular clinical logic, and that in turn this is perpetuated by lack of knowledge and scientific support for psychosocial interventions. Bird *et al.* also caution against complete cessation of such medication in addressing challenging behaviour. Their study shows that the primary route to addressing an individual presenting with this behaviour is to look beyond the behaviour to the cause (the underlying need) and to work with this, which may include the use of some psychotropic medication. In this instance the coordination of psychosocial responses together with psychotropic medication must be tailored to the individual on a case-by-case basis.

What becomes apparent given the range of possible explanations for behaviour termed challenging that Stokes (2000) describes is that there are potentially a multitude of factors involved in providing an explanation for an individual's behaviour. These factors are a composite of individual make-up, the character and life experiences of the person, the effects of dementia on that individual, the context of their current life, where they live and with whom and the characteristics and responses of those significant in the individual's daily life. What is required is an approach that can gather information on all of these factors in order to provide an explanation for the individual's behaviour. What we are striving to identify is why this person behaves in this way at this time and what might they be trying to communicate. In this way we can then hypothesise on why the individual is behaving in the way they are and speculate on what the underlying need might be. From that point we can plan changes to our behaviour and the environment to ensure the underlying need is met. We must also be open to the notion that this will often be a process of trial and error as we seek the changes that will best suit the individual. Bird *et al.* (2002) describe this process as 'an information gathering and hypothesis testing approach to patients and their idiosyncratic difficulties and, secondly, application of a package of interventions which best fit the case profile built from that information'. They state that assessment is the key element in this process. Assessment will seek to describe the behaviour, the circumstances under which it occurs and importantly the circumstances when it does not occur. This assessment should be undertaken through discussion with all those involved in the caring relationship. This may include staff in institutional settings, family and the person themselves. Staff should consider whether the way they undertake care practice could be contributing to the behaviour and notice whether certain staff experience more or less of the behaviour during their care experiences. For example, does one member of staff always experience an aggressive response when helping the individual to use the toilet while another rarely experiences an aggressive response? The staff member experiencing less aggression is likely to have developed an understanding of the individual's underlying need, together with ways of meeting that need which, if shared with other carers, could enable all care team members to care in a way that responds to the individual's underlying need, thus negating the need for the person to exhibit challenging behaviour.

Once the behaviour is described and the circumstances under which it is evident are known, staff can consider (a) what the individual might be trying to communicate and (b) what could be done differently that might decrease the need for the individual to behave in a challenging way. This is the stage that Bird *et al.* term 'hypothesis testing', as carers try out different ways of responding to the individual when they are likely to exhibit challenging behaviour.

Family involvement in the assessment can shed light on an individual's behaviour from the perspective of their life history and personality. This information should be added to the observations and knowledge of the individual that have been gathered and utilised to further inform the assessment and care planning process.

Taking a slightly different approach, Foley *et al.* (2003) sought to establish which of the nonpharmacological techniques employed by staff at specialist continuing care units produced success in managing problematic behaviour. They found that staff used multiple techniques, including activities, interpersonal approaches, physical restraint, reducing stimuli and punishment or force. Of these techniques those associated with successful management were activities and interpersonal approaches. These psychosocial approaches included using redirection, providing one-to-one care, using validation and being flexible in meeting individual's needs. These positive approaches also involved the use of humour, persistence, charting behaviours, involving more staff, being attentive, using the individual's name and being affectionate. They found that the use of restraint and psychotropic medications were associated with failure to successfully manage problematic behaviour.

They further identified that recognising and treating a physical or medical symptom was associated with greater degrees of success. This could be something as simple as identifying that the individual was in pain and providing pain relief. It is also important to assess for depression, particularly as patients with a coexisting depression have been found to exhibit more challenging behaviours than patients with fewer symptoms of depression (Harper *et al.* 2004). Foley *et al.* found that positive involvement of family carers increased the likelihood of successful management of challenging behaviour. Such involvement included frequent visiting, problem solving with staff, providing life history details, giving information on likes and dislikes, contributing to decision making and carrying out caring activities. Conversely, where family carers were unsupportive or behaved contrary to agreed plans, there was an increased likelihood of management being unsuccessful. What was also apparent was that the most difficult behaviours to manage were unpredictable aggression and those behaviours associated with psychiatric comorbidity, where it was difficult for staff to identify triggers for the behaviour.

What is apparent in recent studies into addressing the needs of people with dementia who behave in challenging ways is that within the health care setting clinicians have multiple skills at their disposal to respond with positive psychosocial interventions. These approaches include ensuring one-to-one time, using empathy, avoiding confrontation, listening to and taking account of what the person with dementia says, providing activities, gathering and using life history information, using touch, using sensitivity during personal care, responding to physical needs, diversion, using music and increasing social interaction time. What appears to be lacking, as Bird *et al.* (2002) identify, is the time to apply the approaches and a system for putting what is known about the individual patient together with a selection of approaches that best fit that individual's needs.

Evidence for Practice

Approaches to Resolve Challenging Behaviour

Assessment of the individual by all those involved in providing care

Assessment to rule out a physical cause (e.g. pain)

A description of the behaviour

A description of circumstances when the behaviour occurs or does not occur

Gathering and attending to information on the individual's life history and personality

Identification of possible needs underlying the behaviour

Responses by the care team that are primarily psychosocial but do not exclude the possibility of using medication, but only where the use of medication is judicious

Application of different approaches in order to establish how the underlying need can be best met for the individual

Approaches that are tailored to the individual

Family contribution and participation

CONCLUSION

The difficulty people with dementia have in controlling language and memory in order to communicate fluently has allowed a culture of denial of their experience to develop and indeed to persist. This is no longer acceptable. Those in caring roles are required to develop methods of communication that enable the person with dementia to express their experience, to give credence to those experiences once expressed and to respond to them. The research is beginning to show that this is possible. The methods of communication the person employs are intrinsically their own, formed from their retained individual abilities, referenced by their life history and in the context of their present circumstances. Successful communication is dependent on the response of the person in receipt of that communication and their ability to recognise an individual's method of communication, work with their retained ability, have knowledge of their life story and pay attention to the circumstances within which the communication occurs.

In reality it matters little how skilled we become at communicating if we continue to deny both ourselves and people with dementia the opportunity to communicate. We must certainly seek research evidence that provides greater clarity about the nature of how the communication of people with dementia is disrupted by dementia. It is not enough to know that individuals have word finding problems or that memory impairment creates difficulties. The research evidence needs to be much more specific before it can truly inform good practice.

The fact that research is not yet able to do this is testament to the complex nature of communication and the fact that communication is much more than the transmission, receipt and interpretation of information. Communication is not a process that can be treated in isolation but is integral to life and life quality as a whole. Communication occurs in the context of relationships – how they are formed and sustained, how people view and present themselves to others and how they are viewed and accepted by others together with the volume and range of opportunities to communicate that exist or that can be created.

Throughout this chapter it has become increasingly clear that communication is important not of itself but for the possibilities it offers individuals to seek and secure social inclusion and confirmation that they are indeed individuals who make a valuable contribution to their social world and that their lives are worth living. The level of communication between individuals reflects the nature of the relationship between them. In dementia care the relationship between the carer and cared for reflects a need to meet the physical care needs of the person with dementia and carers seek to refine and employ techniques in communication that enable those physical care needs to be addressed. The research strongly suggests that once this is achieved and, as Ward *et al.* (2005) identify, the person is enabled to get out of bed, wash, dress, eat and drink, use the toilet and return to bed, the requirement for communication is met and further communication is largely considered not needed and therefore is not offered.

Setterlund (1998) identifies that a change in the focus of care occurs when the person with dementia moves from family to institutional care. In so doing they move from care that is informed by a relationship to care that is task-based and stems from acute models of care. Nolan *et al.* (1995) assert that care stemming from acute care models which seek cure, treatment or rehabilitation are inappropriate models for dementia care. It is more appropriate that the focus of care in the specialism should be on supporting an individual's self-esteem needs and that the aim, where a return to former functioning is no longer possible, should be 'actively to develop new and, if possible, equally valued roles and functions which maintain the self esteem of the older person'. They conclude that a meaningful relationship is the crux of good nursing care, particularly in the continuing care environment, and cite Ruddock (1969) who identified that individuals need their existence to be of some significance and the need to have enduring relationships was more important than the need to survive. It could be argued that care offered in institutional settings has made good inroads into enabling people with dementia to survive for longer, but possibly at the expense of the more important needs to lead an existence within which the individual is of some significance and has enduring relationships.

Over the past 15 years there has been a growing interest in questioning the focus of care in the specialism and there is now a strong suggestion that caring for people with dementia amounts to much more than the meeting of physical care needs and that indeed rather than concentrating on quality of *care* we should in fact be more concerned about quality of *life* for the individual. The elements that quality of life focused care should consider and the manner in which communication can support these elements are considered in Chapter 7.

The significance of getting this aspect of dementia care right is momentous. The research highlights the importance of sustaining communication with people with dementia at all stages of the disease; to do so will ensure their continued influence on their own lives. Whether the communication is used to redesign existing services or to ensure the service is tweaked to meet the individual's requirements or to provide crucial social contact that maintains a sense of self, or indeed all of the above, it is a key element to effective care and good life quality.

7 Putting Quality into a Life Lived with Dementia

INTRODUCTION

When considering the advent of person centred care in Chapter 3 we saw that adopting a medical approach to care leads practitioners to seek treatment and cure and to manage problem behaviour. The proposal under person centred care is that the individual's social psychology cannot be detached from their experience of dementia and that the meeting of psychological needs is paramount. In pursuit of a person centred approach there is now consensus that the focus of care should be on improving the quality of life of persons living with dementia. In Chapter 6 we began to appreciate the importance of communication in relation to supporting personhood and meeting psychological needs. We identified that, particularly within institutional care settings, opportunities for people with dementia to communicate are largely concentrated during times when carers undertake physical care and that this represents only a minuscule proportion of the individual's day. We got a sense also that although research is offering some fine examples of how to communicate effectively with people with dementia there are no specific guidelines or principles that can be employed to bring about effective communication. What we are coming to understand is that, as Allan (2001) identifies with respect to the communication needs of people with dementia, certain approaches work for certain individuals at certain times and under certain circumstances.

We are required to respond to people with dementia taking these factors into account, but are required also to give serious consideration to the opportunities we provide that will support and encourage the employment of our communication skills. What is the point of becoming specialist communicators if we do not create opportunities for that communication to take place? We should apply our communication then in relationships that seek to meet not only the individual's physical needs but more importantly their psychosocial needs, for it is through the meeting of these needs that life quality may be determined and a life lived with dementia may be considered worth living.

Many texts, research studies and anecdotal works refer to quality of life and activities to promote quality of life for people who have dementia without actually defining what quality of life might constitute with dementia. This chapter begins by attempting to redress this oversight by examining what is meant by quality of life and the factors considered important to ensure life is worth living from the perspective of a person with dementia. We will then consider how these factors can be used to define objectives for carers to not only sustain but improve the quality of life of persons living with dementia. The chapter also includes a discussion of how the meeting of these objectives may be pursued by clinicians.

QUALITY OF LIFE WITH DEMENTIA

Research into quality of life (QOL), what constitutes QOL, who has it and what influences it is an area of interest in numerous fields. *The Economist* Intelligence Unit's Quality-of-Life Index (2005) gives nine factors that determine life satisfaction: material well-being, health, political stability and security, family life, community life, climate and geography, job security, political freedom and gender equality. Galloway (2006) states that discourse on QOL has existed since the time of Aristotle and that much of the current debate on QOL is found in the literature of the health care sector, where QOL proves a difficult concept to define and where many articles about QOL do not define the concept at all.

A definition by Koot (2001) appears to encompass all the aspects considered relevant when he describes QOL as 'the combination of objectively and subjectively indicated well-being in multiple domains of life considered salient in one's culture and time, while adhering to universal standards of human rights'. This definition recognises that there are both subjective and objective measures of QOL and the importance of an individual's particular situation, background and history, together with the factors generally agreed as important human opportunities.

There has long been interest in investigating how health and ill-health affect an individual's QOL. This interest stems from a desire to identify the factors associated with a particular disease or syndrome that reduces QOL for the person with it, because once these factors are defined steps can be taken to counteract their influence and improve QOL. In chronic disease states where those providing care services are unlikely to be able to influence the progress or outcome of the disease, concentrating on the factors that influence QOL is considered very important. In many chronic disease specialties research has contributed to the definition of QOL, identification of domains relevant to QOL with the specified disease and tools to measure QOL, which in turn serve as outcome measures for evaluating the effectiveness of care practices and drug treatments. Of course, as with many areas of research into dementia, the contribution by research into QOL with dementia is both relatively new and relatively sparse, but is desperately needed to propel practice forward.

Brod *et al.* (1999) point out that QOL in dementia needs to be described and understood, not only so that the effectiveness of service programmes can be evaluated and the efficacy of drug treatments can be tested but also to contribute to the ethical debate regarding health care resource allocation, to aid end of life decision making and to enable the development of clinical guidelines. Already this research is beginning to raise issues for practitioners; for example, the way in which QOL is assessed in relation to the provision of antidementia drugs is being called into question. The premise of the effectiveness of these drugs is that they improve cognition and so benefit QOL, but research undertaken by Banerjee *et al.* (2006) has discovered that cognition is not a key determinant in QOL for people with dementia. The National Institute for Health and Clinical Excellence, as the government agency charged with determining the cost effectiveness of drugs such as Donepzil, Galatamine, Rivastigmine and Memantine and the availability of these drugs to the majority of people, is coming under increased pressure to broaden the definition of QOL in dementia and to take other factors into account when making decisions about the effectiveness of these drugs.

Another key motivation for describing QOL for someone with dementia is that if we understand the aspects that determine QOL for an individual with dementia it should prevent others, carers included, from speculating on how poor QOL must be for a person with dementia. We make judgements from our healthy perspective, and it must be admitted that most healthy people, particularly young people, see death as preferable to dementia. Patrick *et al.* (1994) confirmed this, demonstrating that both dementia and coma were considered states compared to which death would be preferable. If we as carers approach people with dementia with the belief that they would be better off dead it will be very difficult for this view not to impact on our caring practices. We are required to acknowledge, as Mack and Whitehouse (2001) point out, that not only do expectations for QOL change with age and health but what seems to provide QOL for a healthy person may change if they develop dementia. Furthermore, as Logsdon *et al.* (2002) state, judgements as to what is important in QOL may change as dementia progresses. What is vital, of course, before we can begin to focus our caring practices towards enabling people with dementia to improve their QOL is that we start from the premise that a good QOL *is* possible when you have dementia.

Bowling *et al.* (2003), in an effort to explore older people's definitions and priorities for a good quality of life for themselves and their peers, interviewed nearly one thousand people over the age of 65. The factors most associated with life quality were judged to be social relationships and health: loss of health was the factor that took QOL away and good social relationships contributed to good QOL. Other important factors included social roles and activities, psychological outlook and well-being, finances, independence and home and neighbourhood.

In attempting to quantify QOL factors for a life lived with dementia many of these factors remain important. Much of the research in this area can be found in the studies seeking to develop a method of measuring QOL of people with dementia. The vast majority of the assessment tools developed bear the influence of Lawton's conceptualisation of QOL (Lawton 1994, 1997; Lawton *et al.* 1999). Assessment of QOL, Lawton argued, should include consideration of both objective and subjective factors and four overarching domains are influential: psychological well-being, behavioural competence, the objective environment and perceived QOL. Many of the commentators considered important in this area of research, including Brod *et al.* (1999), Rabins (1999), Logsdon *et al.* (2002), Ready *et al.* (2002) and Tester *et al.* (2003), identify similar sets of components that are considered to be relevant in respect of QOL lived with dementia. Drawing from the work of these commentators, a list has been provided of the factors considered most important in QOL with dementia (see below). It should be remembered that the weight of importance attached to each factor will vary, depending on individual needs, desires and circumstances.

Evidence for Practice

Factors Considered Important in QOL with Dementia

To have a sense of self

To interact socially and to be involved in relationships

To be actively involved in meaningful and enjoyable activities

To be subjectively satisfied with life in general and to experience a sense of well-being

To be able to influence what happens to one and the surroundings

To be able to undertake the basic activities required for daily living

To be physically healthy

Tester *et al.* (2003) observed that the subjects of their study, frail older people (half of whom had dementia), not only perceived that they had a good QOL but were also actively attempting to improve their QOL. This would imply that the onus is on those around the individual, particularly those charged with a caring role, to recognise the potential for maintaining and improving QOL and to identify and operationalise the skills and opportunities that need to exist for this to happen. Considering the factors listed as influential in QOL with dementia, we can describe a further list of objectives for carers in pursuit of supporting and improving life quality for people with dementia.

Evidence for Practice

Carers' Objectives to Support QOL for Persons with Dementia

To be proactive in supporting persons with dementia in maintaining their sense of who they are

To be proactive in providing opportunity and specialist support to ensure that the person with dementia is enabled to remain engaged in social activity and relationships, both existing and new

To be proactive in providing opportunity and specialist support for the person with dementia to be involved in activity and occupation that is meaningful and enjoyable

To monitor, evaluate and be responsive to the individual's subjective satisfaction with life

To consult actively with the person with dementia on an ongoing basis to ensure that they are influential in what happens to and around them

To ensure optimum independence in undertaking activities of daily living on the part of the person with dementia

To ensure the individual experiences the optimum physical health possible for them

The good news, from the carer's perspective, is that the factors associated with QOL are tangibly conditional upon one another, so attending to one area will have an impact on the others. Therefore if carers develop relationships with the person with dementia and involve them in meaningful occupation then their sense of self and esteem will be supported. When the sense of self and esteem are increased the individual will feel confident in their ability to attempt to influence their environment. Similarly, it is a condition of a meaningful relationship that the emotional well-being of those in the relationship is important and any distress or emotional discomfort is recognised and attended to. The bad news for individuals with dementia is that where carers are ignorant of these factors or fail to attend to them QOL is likely to be extremely poor.

It is beyond the scope of this book to investigate and describe in detail how the carers' objectives identified above can be operationalised, but a preliminary consideration is possible and is described below.

TO BE PROACTIVE IN SUPPORTING PERSONS WITH DEMENTIA IN MAINTAINING THEIR SENSE OF WHO THEY ARE

This will involve getting to know the person as an individual and reinforcing their individuality and identity during each interaction. It is reflected in actions as simple as using the person's preferred name, surrounding them with familiar things, knowing and applying personal preferences and ensuring access to people important to them. Contact with people who know the individual well and who have biographical detail, family and friends in particular, will not only reinforce the person's identity, the context of their lives and their continued importance to their immediate community but also enable staff in caring institutions to use the personal information provided by intimates to know the individual better, so that they can then utilise information in a positive manner to support self-awareness and esteem.

Similarly, it is important that the person is encouraged and enabled to remain involved in activities and community resources that are important to them, such as attending a familiar place of worship or continuing to attend accustomed social events or hobbies. Traditionally, where maintaining this activity becomes problematic the activity may be replaced by something similar within the person's own home or the home they live in; for example, where church attendance is problematic the vicar may undertake regular home visits or going out to a tea dance may be replaced by listening to music at home or a dance organised at the nursing home. The arrangement of such activities seeks to address the underlying needs, in the example cases, for spiritual expression and social activity, and as such is appropriate. However, in settling for an approximation of the accustomed activity an opportunity to have a sense of self and identity doubly reinforced is undoubtedly lost. At some point this may have to happen anyway, if the individual's dementia progresses such that usual activity cannot be sustained. However, we should be aware that in replacing a usual activity something is lost and efforts to sustain accustomed activity in the accustomed manner should be significant.

The evidence for life story work, reminiscence and memory books supports such activity as being useful in both increasing carers' knowledge of the person and in supporting a sense of self. Our communication with the person should reinforce who they are, re-telling stories that involved the person, reminding them what they have done with their lives, the history they have lived through, their contribution to it and to the lives of their families and communities. If, as Sabat (2002) holds, our sense of who we are is dependent on the acknowledgement of this and the reinforcement of this by those around us, then as carers of people who have dementia a key undertaking of the caring role must be taking responsibility for acknowledging and reinforcing identity throughout our interaction. It is particularly important that those caring in institutional settings, such as hospital or nursing homes, take up this objective, for frequently in such settings they are the only people around the person with dementia for prolonged periods of time. They must do it because there is no one else to do it.

TO BE PROACTIVE IN PROVIDING OPPORTUNITY AND SPECIALIST SUPPORT TO ENSURE THAT THE PERSON WITH DEMENTIA IS ENABLED TO REMAIN ENGAGED IN SOCIAL ACTIVITY AND RELATIONSHIPS, BOTH EXISTING AND NEW

This objective will be supported by encouraging regular contact with people and social activity important to the person with dementia. It requires that the person is enabled to overcome barriers that dementia brings which undermine the maintenance of relationships and the development of new ones, not only the communication difficulties but stigma, loss of confidence and practical considerations such as accessing social occasions. There is a need in institutional settings for carers to take responsibility for dismantling the organisational barriers that inhibit social engagement and relationships. For most people with dementia being confined to a nursing home restricts the number of opportunities they will have for interaction. Their inability to initiate and sustain conversation limits the likelihood of peer relationships developing within nursing home environments, where something as simple as aligning chairs along a wall can prohibit eye contact and the use of gesture and facial expression that might reflect someone's interest in having a conversation with another.

Carers, professional as well as familial, are required to be available in relationships, to be interested in and to care for the person and to demonstrate that interest and the person's worthiness of that care during every interaction. Forming, sustaining and growing relationships takes time and this time has to be made available. This will not be possible if carers persist in believing that persons with dementia are of less value than others, as we saw in Chapter 3.

Allowing the relationship to be reciprocal and letting the person show their affection for you will also be important. Consider the factors important in most relationships: trust, consistency and affection. These all have a place in our relationships with people with dementia. If they are to be meaningful relationships we must expect them to cost us something emotionally; truthfully, we have to expect that our relationships with a person with dementia will cost us more emotionally, because the nature of dementia means that we must work hard and employ special skills to be in the relationship.

PROVIDING THE OPPORTUNITY AND SPECIALIST SUPPORT TO BE INVOLVED IN MEANINGFUL OCCUPATION AND ACTIVITY

An activity or occupation may be described as 'meaningful' when the desire of the individual to be involved in the activity is matched by their ability to achieve it. The occupation is then 'meaningful' because sense of self, self-esteem and enjoyment are maximised. The skill of the person providing an opportunity for meaningful activity for individuals with dementia lies in knowing the person, knowing their abilities, having the skill to maximise their ability, communicating with them to establish what they find enjoyable and translating that knowledge into an activity that can be accomplished, while ensuring that the time and resources to undertake the activity are available. This is not a one-off process and is likely to involve a degree of trial and error. It is also a process that requires different approaches and different skills depending on the severity of dementia that the individual is experiencing.

Perrin (1997) provides a summary of the effects of activity and inactivity, including the effects on people with dementia. Inactivity is found to lead to decreased alertness, reduced ability to concentrate, increased irritability, increased anxiety, depression, feelings of oppression, problem-solving difficulties and confusion and disorientation. Many of these outcomes of inactivity are recognisable as clinical symptoms of dementia. We may come to one of two conclusions: firstly, inactivity exacerbates dementia symptoms or, secondly, inactivity *causes* dementia symptoms. Perrin also illustrates the psychological benefits that accompany the provision of activity, including an increase in smiling, laughing and talking, an increase in attempts to initiate and engage in social interaction, increased alertness, improvement in memory and concentration, increased expression of emotion and a decrease in agitation. From this perspective the value of ensuring that activity is provided for people who have dementia becomes very important and it is clear to see how meaningful activity contributes to enjoyment of life.

In order to provide the opportunity and support for an individual with dementia to participate and benefit from activity, consideration must be given to the person's ability and skills, what they are likely or known to enjoy and what the level of challenge should be so that the activity is easy enough to achieve but hard enough to be testing, thus avoiding failure and boredom. Knowledge of the person's life history will help us know what they are likely to find interesting and enjoyable, but equally knowing the person as they are now can help us to identify what would now give them pleasure.

For individuals with mild dementia who live at home and are struggling to partici- pate in their accustomed activities the focus of intervention may be twofold: firstly, to support involvement and continued achievement and, secondly, if necessary, finding meaningful replacements. Considering the discussions in previous chapters about the pervasive nature of dementia and accompanying sense of loss many people expe- rience during the early stages, it must be considered that activity that provides an opportunity to come to terms with the diagnosis and to plan for the future are likely to be important for the individual with mild dementia.

Another key factor to consider in relation to activity and early stage dementia is the research currently being generated concerning the benefits of cognitive stimulation therapy (CST). Spector *et al.* (2003) found that a group programme for people with mild to moderate dementia based on stimulating cognition had benefits not only for cognition but also on QOL. The activities undertaken in CST groups for people with dementia include: physical games, number and word games, reminiscence, creative activity, using money and quizzes. The aim of cognitive stimulation activity is to en- able learning and strengthen the individual's existing resources. More recent research by Knapp *et al.* (2006) indicates that not only is this therapeutic activity effective but it is equally as effective as antidementia drugs. The opportunity to be involved in activity that is proven in strengthening personal resources and that acknowledges what is happening to the individual while enabling life quality to be improved will certainly be meaningful for individuals with mild to moderate dementia.

However, the real difficulties in providing meaningful activity for people with dementia occur when an individual moves into the 24-hour care setting, because it is at this point that the person's difficulty in seeking and maintaining accustomed activity is most likely to be met by the inability of the care setting to either recognise or respond to this difficulty, and to be exacerbated by poor understanding of the benefits of activity and detriments of inactivity. We have seen in previous chapters how the organisation of care environments and the pressure on time militates heavily against the provision of opportunities for meaningful occupation.

Perrin (2005) identifies a further significant organisational barrier to the provision of meaningful activity for people with dementia, that of the culture of the organisation. Cultures are underpinned by beliefs and it follows that, according to Perrin, the activity culture will be driven by beliefs held about activities. If the belief is that activity is pointless and of less value than other organisational tasks and those cared for are believed to be incapable of participating in activity, then it is unlikely that activity will be given any priority and may in fact not take place at all. Further, Perrin identifies, where a member of staff does attempt to conduct activities their efforts are likely to be undermined by others within the environment. Perrin (2005) identifies three conditions of effective activity provision in care settings: firstly, belief that activity has the potential to improve a person's health, secondly, an understanding of the relationship between activity and health and inactivity and ill-health and, finally, demonstrable evidence of the capacity for activity to bring positive changes to a person's well-being. The role of the manager in care settings is crucial to the successful implementation of activity and the priority given to it. If the person in charge does not support and embed a culture that recognises and supports the importance of activity and the need to be occupied there is little hope of such a culture prevailing.

The ideal approach to activity provision is that it is person centred, based on an individual assessment of what will work for that person and contributes to their well-being. At times this will be a solitary or one-to-one activity and at times it will be a group-based activity. Working with people in groups has many benefits; it provides group members with the opportunity to have social contact, to form and maintain relationships and to have self-awareness, esteem and identity supported.

Working with groups can also provide a way in which the occupation and activity needs of people can be addressed in a less resource intensive manner than one-to-one activity. There is a rich history of such groupwork for people for dementia in day services, which could be transferred to 24-hour care environments. Many books have been published on groupwork for people with dementia that demonstrate how the needs of the individual and their QOL can be supported through such work; examples include Dent (2003), Bender (2004) and Perrin (2004).

The benefits to carers of providing, supporting and participating in meaningful activities with people who have dementia is a grossly under-researched area, but anecdotal and experiential evidence tell us that satisfaction with work is improved and relationships with people with dementia enhanced. If this proves to be true then there are further important reasons for ensuring people with dementia are supported in their involvement in meaningful activity. Job satisfaction is highly correlated to low rates of absenteeism and low staff turnover, both particular problems in long term dementia care.

TO MONITOR, EVALUATE AND BE RESPONSIVE TO THE INDIVIDUAL'S SUBJECTIVE SATISFACTION WITH LIFE

We have already seen that much of the literature concerning QOL and people with dementia is found in research into the manner in which QOL can be assessed and the validation of tools to measure QOL in dementia. These tools represent formal ways to monitor and evaluate QOL in persons with dementia. Three methods have been identified to accomplish such evaluation: firstly, self-report by the person with dementia, most often relied upon when the person is judged to have the communication skills to verbalise their satisfaction with life; secondly, proxy reports, usually made by informal carers; thirdly, judgements made following observations by trained observers. Although some researchers have chosen to use a combination of methods, the most commonly used and widely recognised, dementia care mapping (DCM), is of the latter variety. DCM has been refined and developed by the Bradford Dementia Group (2005) as a tool to assess the quality of care and improve QOL in 24-hour care settings. Kitwood (1997) described DCM as 'a serious attempt to take the standpoint of the person with dementia, using a combination of empathy and observational skill'. DCM has long held a strong role in providing information on an individual's response to the factors associated with QOL and thus can offer important information to enable care practices to be honed to suit individual needs, even where barriers to communication are strongly in evidence. Brooker (2005) provides a review of the nature of DCM as a tool and its efficacy.

Other scales developed to measure QOL in dementia include the dementia quality of life instrument (Brod *et al.* 1999), a tool that relies on the perspective of the person with dementia and is most appropriate for use with individuals in the mild to moderate stages of dementia, the Cornell Brown Scale for Quality of Life (Ready *et al.* 2002), which includes perspectives of both the carer and person with dementia and is used primarily with individuals with mild to moderate dementia, and the quality of life in late-stage dementia (Weiner *et al.* 2000), designed to measure QOL of individuals with advanced dementia in institutional settings. An overview of the QOL measures for dementia currently in use is provided by Ready and Ott (2003).

It is encouraging that interest in developing methods of measuring QOL of people with dementia is growing. The ability to measure the effectiveness of care interventions and treatments will enable the cycle of improvement. Once we can measure the effectiveness of what we are doing we can identify what is ineffective and act to remedy this, measure again and so the cycle is stimulated. What is required of practitioners is that they become familiar with the factors associated with QOL, both in broad terms and in terms of what is important to the individual, and then to familiarise themselves with validated tools and to use them to make an assessment of QOL of individuals in their care, with the primary goal of improving QOL for those individuals.

TO CONSULT ACTIVELY WITH THE PERSON WITH DEMENTIA ON AN ONGOING BASIS TO ENSURE THAT THEY ARE INFLUENTIAL IN WHAT HAPPENS TO AND AROUND THEM

One of the huge strides forward that has been achieved in dementia care over the past decade is the growing awareness that it is possible to consult with people with dementia and to sustain consultation throughout the course of a life lived with dementia. In Chapter 5 we saw how evidence from Miesen (1997), Tappen *et al.* (1999), Ostwald *et al.* (2002) and Sabat (2002), among others, illuminated our understanding that people with dementia, even advanced dementia, retain awareness of their illness and its effects and can communicate this awareness. Indeed, it is this communication and our developing ability to access and sustain this communication that is informing our current understanding of what it is like to live with dementia.

Consultation with and the empowerment of people with dementia has one main aim, to enable people with dementia to influence their own lives. This aim can be realised in terms of groups of people living with dementia, by promoting and providing opportunities for people with dementia to express their thoughts and opinions on national and local policy with regard to health and social care provision. Similarly, by listening to individual opinions and preferences on a day-to-day basis and incorporating these into the plans of care we develop with them, we may ensure their continued ability to influence their own everyday life.

There is a need to ensure that for individuals living with dementia, one of the most important means of demonstrating and practising a person centred approach is through continuous consultation with and the involvement of the individual in the decisions that are taken about their lives.

If we are to actively consult with people with dementia this consultation needs to commence when our contact with them commences, which ideally begins at the point of diagnosis. In an ideal world, following early diagnosis there would be sensitive disclosure with supportive follow-up, the individual would be involved in planning for their future and would be the controlling partner in any caring relationship. The key to such endeavours will lie in communication, our ability to communicate in a manner accessible to the person and our ability to interpret and be responsive to their communication.

Consultation and the facilitation of choice can be a large undertaking, such as an advance directive to refuse resuscitation in the event of cardiac arrest or a small undertaking such as what to eat for lunch. The skill for carers is in understanding that the size of the decision to be taken in relation to the involvement of the person the decision will affect is equal. Whether the decision is huge and life changing or small and life enhancing is not the most important aspect, which is to recognise the individual's right to be involved in and supported in making the decision. The right to choice and involvement in decision making is not simply a matter of choice but of the importance placed on the person's involvement. Denying the right of the person to be consulted indicates that the person's opinion is not respected; such exclusion goes against the philosophy of a person centred approach.

Research is showing that consultation is possible throughout the course of dementia. It is beginning to describe the nature of the processes and skills that will be required to initiate and sustain consultation. There is a requirement then that as carers we fully accept that consultation is possible, and develop ways of initiating and sustaining consultation and integrating consultation into daily practice.

However, in order to fulfil this objective and to enhance QOL of people living with dementia it is not enough to undertake consultation; there must be action following consultation. If we consult with and gather the opinions, desires and complaints of people with dementia as a group or on an individual basis we must ensure that the services we offer in response are reactive to the opinions, desires and complaints expressed. Then we will be making progress in enabling people with dementia to remain in control of what happens to them and to remain influential in terms of what happens to and around them.

TO ENSURE OPTIMUM INDEPENDENCE IN UNDERTAKING ACTIVITIES OF DAILY LIVING ON THE PART OF THE PERSON WITH DEMENTIA

The activities that an individual undertakes throughout the day to manage their lives can be loosely divided into instrumental activities of daily living (IADL) and self-care activities of daily living (ADL). Lawton and Brody (1969) define the IADL as the ability to use the telephone, ability to use transport to get around, ability to shop, ability to complete laundry, ability to take responsibility for own medication, ability to manage finances, ability to prepare meals and ability to perform household tasks. Self-care ADL refer to the abilities in bathing, using the toilet, dressing, remaining continent, transferring and feeding (Katz *et al.* 1970). The pattern of impairment in dementia means that an individual is likely to experience difficulty with IADL from an early point, with increasing difficulty in performing self-care ADL as dementia progresses. For the individual the prospect of dependence on others from the onset of dementia is real.

A study conducted by Anderson *et al.* (2004) found that dependency upon others to perform activities of daily living was the main factor affecting QOL for persons with dementia. This finding underlines the importance of developing partnerships with people with dementia that recognise that prolonging independence will enhance QOL. In order to be effective in working with individuals to prolong independence clinicians will need to work with the person to establish what is threatening or compromising their independence and to find a strategy that will enable that individual to overcome the difficulty. One of the advantages of involving individuals with dementia in support groups is that these groups provide a means of sharing information and advice that can enable the individual to maximise their independence, by learning from others living with dementia and from professionals with experience of helping individuals with dementia. Simple tips like the use of diaries, calendars, notes, computers, paying bills by direct debit, considering power of attorney, introducing routine into daily and weekly life and making specific plans to counteract common problems can have enormous benefits in enhancing independence.

The use of technology in supporting independence in people with dementia is a growing area of interest and research. One example, the Enable Project, established in 2001, set out to study the use of technological devices by people with dementia with the specific aim of promoting independence and enabling people to manage daily tasks for themselves. Reports from several European countries (available at http://www.enableproject.org/index.html) reflect positive outcomes in using technological devices, including increased independence, improved QOL, enhanced sense of empowerment and increased safety. Among the devices tested were an automatic day and night calendar, an automatic bedroom lamp which is activated when a person gets out of bed, a lost item locater, time orientation devices, a gas cooker monitor, a medicine reminder and a picture phone. A further finding of the project is that for the person to gain maximum benefit from the devices they need, usage should begin as early as possible so that the person can get used to the technology and its use becomes habitual.

There is much that can be done to enable people with dementia to remain in their own homes and to manage their lives with a good degree of independence, but there will always be a balance to be struck between enabling someone to live independently and ensuring their safety. At some point it may become clear that the balance between independence and safety can no longer be achieved and risks become too high for the individual to remain safely within their own home. Therefore a move into 24-hour care becomes unavoidable, but it is vital at this point to remember that working to prolong independence should continue.

The strictures already described of living with dementia in many 24-hour care settings mean that the pressure of time frequently leads to carers completing tasks for the person rather than facilitating their doing things for themselves. Those with experience of completing personal care and dressing tasks for others will know that in the majority of cases washing and dressing someone else is not only speedier than waiting and encouraging them to do it for themselves but the end result is often more presentable, in the view of the person undertaking the task at any rate. Moving someone using a wheelchair is certainly quicker than escorting someone who is slow to walk or needs the physical support of others. However, we should no longer focus on providing care for the benefit of the organisation, or indeed the carer, but should be concerned with enhancing the life quality of the person with dementia, so activity that centres on extending independence is necessary.

The skills required of carers are that they recognise and prompt the skills and abilities the person has and where they cannot be enabled to complete tasks fully independently their participation in as far as is possible is fostered. If we consider the features of dementia that make undertaking washing and dressing activities difficult we can begin to examine these activities and to understand how they can be made achievable. For example, an individual may not be able to locate and select the clothing they need to dress when faced with the challenge of finding the cupboards the clothes are kept in, choosing from a large selection and ensuring all the required items are assembled and put on in the correct order, but they may be able to dress independently if clothes are laid out in order or passed to them one at a time. Verbal and physical prompts can also help. It is difficult to prescribe a full list of what can enable individuals in self-care activities simply because for each person the difficulty and the solution are likely to be individual and so require investigation and negotiation between carer and the person with dementia. There is often a fine line between encouraging independence and causing the person stress because an activity is beyond their ability. What is certain is that for each person in all activities there is a position between leaving the person to their own devices and failure and doing everything for them that represents their optimum level of functional ability. Finding this optimum level is the goal of the carer; the outcome of doing so is enhanced QOL.

The progress made in developing the design of environments for people with dementia that maximise their functional ability has been great over the past 10 years. Tombs (1997) identifies five principles underpinning design of environments for people who have dementia: buildings need to make sense so that persons with dementia can quickly understand them, they should help the person to find their way about, the environment should be therapeutic, it should be safe and it should be a quality environment.

It is now possible to build environments that help the person to make sense of where they are, to locate rooms, to identify the purpose of the rooms and to locate and use items within rooms appropriately. The use of signage and colour to highlight areas and items to enable independence in the use of the toilet, kitchen, bathroom or bedroom areas is growing. Simple measures could be constructing storage areas without doors or kitchen cupboards with see through doors so that items stored are easily identifiable. We are also realising with respect to design that traditional-looking appliances such as toilet flushes, toilet roll holders, light switches and clocks with hands and numbers are easier for people with dementia to recognise and interpret than many labour saving modern design items such as digital clocks or taps that are activated by passing a hand in front of a sensor, which prove confusing and difficult to use when you have dementia.

There is no doubt that design and technology will continue to develop apace and provide new ways of enhancing independence in both IADL and self-care ADL for people with dementia. The level of consultation and the nature of the relationship between people with dementia and clinicians will be instrumental in determining how optimum independence in undertaking activities of daily life will be achieved for each individual living with dementia. However, it is necessary for many clinicians, particularly those working in institutional care, to begin to view care not as an activity that involves doing something but rather an activity that encourages individuals to do things for themselves for as long as possible. What many clinicians might find is that this is a much more enjoyable, albeit time consuming, method of practising caring.

ATTEND TO PHYSICAL HEALTH NEEDS

We have already considered some of the aspects pertinent to the physical health needs of people with dementia. It is worth reiterating that a diagnosis of dementia neither precludes the possibility of other health problems nor negates the need for treatment, and this remains true throughout the person's life with dementia and is not relevant at the point of establishing a diagnosis only. One of the pieces of advice that has long been part of dementia care training is that any change in behaviour or level of need on the part of the person may be the result of a physical health problem as yet undiagnosed; infection, injury, constipation and pressure sores are the most commonly cited. Although much of the advice given with regard to the care of persons with dementia that is more than 15 years old should now be discarded, this should not.

While the traditional approach to health problems in people with dementia urges carers to identify and respond to any symptoms exhibited, what we are beginning to discover is that there is much more we can do in respect of healthy living for people who develop dementia. People who develop dementia related to vascular disease and strokes can benefit from advice regarding diet, exercise and smoking, and health promotion aimed at older adults, for those over 65, is no less relevant because someone has dementia. Indeed, health promotion in this case is likely to require specific skills of carers to ensure people with dementia have the optimum opportunity to avail themselves of the advice.

It is certainly worth considering with regard to the physical health of people with dementia the way in which challenge to the accepted knowledge can bring positive change. For example, a study by Biernacki and Barratt (2001) revealed that nutritional problems, rather than being symptomatic of dementia and irreversible, are the consequence of the effects of dementia and are open to care interventions that not only ensure adequate and enjoyable nutrition but also contribute to an improved sense of well-being and life quality. The study also demonstrated the advantages of looking to other disciplines to contribute their knowledge and expertise to the care of people with dementia.

The dementia multidisciplinary care team has traditionally comprised registered mental nurses, social workers, psychiatrists and occupational therapists. However, over the past 10 years the involvement of less traditional allied health professionals in the care of people with dementia has demonstrated significant progress in advancing care practice in specific health areas. The Biernacki and Barratt study describes how the combined skills of nursing, dietetics, speech and language therapy, psychology, occupational therapy, catering and pharmacy can overcome the nutritional problems associated with advanced dementia. This line of thought is pursued in Chapter 9, where the care of people with advanced dementia and the potential role of palliative specialists are discussed.

The objective of meeting the physical health needs of people with dementia has the potential to be much more than a response to observed signs and symptoms of ill-health; it has the potential to be a proactive and dynamic activity in the sense of health promotion and in incorporating skills, ideas and knowledge from other disciplines and specialist areas to challenge what is the accepted progress and outcome of dementia.

THE ROLE OF COMMUNICATION

In considering how the objectives to support QOL for people with dementia may be met, there is a repeated need to refer to the relationship between the person and the carer and the nature of the consultation between them. Establishing and maintaining communication throughout the course of dementia is vital. Tester *et al.* (2003) confirm the importance of communication in relation to QOL. In their study they found that: 'Communication was a key theme. Being able or enabled to communicate verbally and non-verbally is essential for frail older people to express themselves, maintain a sense of self, form and maintain relationships, participate in interaction and activities, and make meaning of their experiences.' The subject of communication was considered at length in the previous chapter and it is worth reiterating that the skills required involve identifying and overcoming the barriers to communication that dementia, organisations and carers themselves create. The role of professional carers in respect of communicating with persons with dementia commences at the point of contact and continues throughout the person's life with dementia. Good communicators are those who take the time to listen and do not give up when understanding or being understood becomes difficult, they know that communication is possible.

Those who refuse to accept that people with dementia continue to attempt communication even in the face of severe disabilities have no hope of deciphering the complex forms of communication they are likely to encounter and as a result should be excluded from positions of influence in the life of the person with dementia. Those who do not know the individual intimately and who lack skills in deciphering meaning in behaviour will undoubtedly struggle to unlock meaning. The conundrum is often that those with intimate knowledge of the individual's life history, like family and those close to the individual are unlikely to be those trained in interpreting behaviour or skilled in communication techniques, and those trained in interpreting behaviour and skilled in communication techniques, as, for example, mental health professionals, are unlikely to have intimate knowledge of the individual's life history. Both elements are important in communicating with people who have dementia, and while each alone will have some success the method that is most supportive of effective communication is a combination of both. It is this level of communication that will support the work of enhancing QOL for persons who have dementia.

CONCLUSION

Medical science and a close traditional alliance of dementia care and a medical perspective has brought dementia care to the point where there is a strong recognition of the need to ensure the safety, nourishment, health and cleanliness of the body, and the possibility of adding years to a life lived with dementia has become a reality. However, given what the research is now revealing in respect of the psychological and social needs of people with dementia, unless there is similarly, a strong recognition and response to these needs we will be guilty of prolonging life at the expense of quality of life. A life lived with dementia where psychosocial needs are unattended is an existence, not a life in the sense one would want to live it. In effect we are now required to add life to years rather than simply adding years to life.

There is enough research to indicate the factors most individuals with dementia consider important to their QOL and information suggesting that people with dementia persist in trying to sustain and improve their QOL. There is also enough information to start to develop ways of practising and working with persons who have dementia and to support them in improving the quality of their lives.

Practitioners are required to understand the factors people with dementia, as a group, specify as impacting on their QOL and also to use methods of communication that facilitate greater understanding of individual nuances so that they can concentrate their caring efforts on improving individual QOL. Initially and most importantly we are required to embrace the knowledge that the quality of a life lived with dementia has the potential not only to be good but to be better.

8   Getting the Most from Drug Treatment

INTRODUCTION

The focus of attention in relation to drug treatments in dementia care over the past 10 years has increasingly been concentrated on issues concerning the availability and effectiveness of the new antidementia treatments for Alzheimer's disease, the so-called acetylcholinesterase inhibitors. However, the issues around pharmaceutical treatment of people with dementia are much broader than this. Discussion of the use of medications in the treatment of older adults is a growing area within health research, and this research is raising serious concerns about the difficulties associated with ensuring that prescribed drug treatments have the desired outcomes with this section of the population, which includes a large proportion of those living with dementia. In the care of people with dementia, as could perhaps be predicted, both the effects of dementia and the attitude and behaviour of health professionals complicate an already complicated issue.

This chapter begins with an examination of the pertinent issues in relation to the prescription of drug treatments for older adults and, more specifically, people who have dementia, and goes on to consider the general principles around the application of pharmaceutical approaches used in dementia care. There is discussion of antidementia drugs and other drug treatments commonly used in dementia care, including the increasingly controversial use of psychotropic medication to control behaviours that challenge the skills of carers.

PHARMACOTHERAPY IN OLDER ADULTS

In terms of the population of the United Kingdom those over 65 years represent 18 % of the total population, yet 45 % of the medication prescribed in the United Kingdom is prescribed for those over 65. The findings of the Health Survey for England (1998) were that four out of five people aged over 75 years take at least one type of medication and that 36 % take four or more preparations, with an average of 22 items dispensed per older adult each year. Several other startling statistics accompany this rate of prescription; up to 50 % of older adults may not be taking medication as prescribed (Marinker 1997), older adults are three times more likely to be admitted to hospital as a result of an adverse reaction to prescribed drugs and

70 to 80 % of prescribed medication is issued through repeat prescription (Hudson & Boyter 1997). These figures begin to hint at the range of difficulties associated with the use of drug therapy in older adults and with people who have dementia, who form a significant proportion of this population, as difficulties are compounded by factors associated with dementia. The main factors for consideration with regard to older adults and prescription medication consist of changes in the way the body uses drugs, concordance issues, polypharmacy and the lack of a systematic review, which leads to reliance on repeat prescriptions.

The manner in which drugs are absorbed, distributed, metabolised and eliminated by the body changes with age. These changes can impact upon the anticipated effect of medication and whether or not the desired outcome may be achieved. A prolonged half-life of drugs (particularly psychotropic preparations) and an increase in the effect of drugs can result, meaning that lower doses are not only safer but frequently adequate in achieving the desired outcome in older adults rather than doses advised for younger adults. The advice commonly offered in relation to medication for older people is to start low and go slow and to recognise that in some individuals the onset of the full therapeutic effect may be delayed and adequate time should be allowed between increases in dosage. In the care of people with dementia this is particularly relevant as the delayed onset of effect may lead to an accumulation of the drug in the body, which may result in behaviour more likely to be interpreted as deterioration due to dementia rather than the effect of prescribed medication. For example, sleeping tablets may have a delayed onset of several hours in older adults. Therefore a younger adult taking the medication at 11 at night may be asleep within an hour; for an older person the effect may be delayed until 3 in the morning. After several days the cumulative effect is likely to be that the older person develops a reversed sleep pattern, which in turn may increase levels of confusion and adversely impact on functional ability. In someone with dementia these symptoms are more likely to be interpreted as dementia than recognised as a drug effect, which in turn may lead to the unnecessary prescription of more medication to try and improve night time sleeping and control behaviour.

Ensuring an individual's agreement and cooperation with any element of planned care is important to the success of that care and where medication forms part of the plan concordance is equally important to success. Prescribed medication is most effective when taken in the prescribed manner – at the right time, in the right dose and by the appropriate route. Failure to do so, as Westbury (2003) cautions, may result in poor management of disease, increased recourse to hospital admission, waste of expensive medication and ultimately in premature death. With an estimated 50 % of older adults failing to take their medication as prescribed there is serious cause for concern. In respect of older adults the presumption is that failure to take medication appropriately is unintentional, that the older person either forgets to take the medication or gets confused and as a result does not take it correctly. Unintentional failure to take medication as prescribed accounts for some of the percentage not doing so; however, it is also true that in common with many presumptions about older people, the presumption that most older adults fail to take medication because they are forgetful or confused proves to be ill founded. Indeed, a study undertaken by Park *et al.* (1999) suggests that older patients make least mistakes when it comes to adhering to their prescribed medication and that it is younger people with busy lifestyles and middle-aged adults who make the most errors. What the research reveals is that rather than failing to comply with medication regimes unintentionally older adults *intentionally* omit to take prescribed medication or take it in a manner other than that advised by the person prescribing. Lowe and Raynor (2000) found that older adults, in common with younger people, made conscious decisions about whether or not to take medication.

There are many reasons why older adults choose not to take their medication: worry about side effects, worry about dependency, concern that the drug is not working, belief that because symptoms have improved the drug is not needed any more and a general dislike for taking tablets. Medication may also be taken at different times to that prescribed as the individual attempts to fit the medication regime into their routine daily life. Medicines may be taken in a manner contrary to that advised; for example, they may be crushed or diluted to aid consumption with poor appreciation of the fact that this may alter the chemical make-up of the preparation. More worryingly, not only do many older adults fail to take, or make adjustment to, medication prescribed for them they do not communicate these self-initiated changes to either the doctor or pharmacist. This will have an impact on the clinician's ability to evaluate the effects of what is prescribed.

The memory difficulty that is a feature of dementia may certainly mean that people with dementia have more difficulty than most in remembering to take medication, to take it at the right time and in the correct manner. However, it would be naïve to presume that people with dementia fail to take medication as prescribed purely because they have dementia. People with dementia may fail to take medicine or change the way in which medicines are taken for exactly the same reasons as people who do not have dementia. Forgetfulness and confusion are not the only factors associated with unintentional nonconcordance. Other factors that may account for unintentional nonconcordance include the inability to read instructions (due to poor eyesight or directions being provided in the wrong language), inability to manipulate containers (particularly childproof bottles or blister packs), poor understanding or misinterpretation of verbal instructions and difficulty managing regimes where more than one medicine is prescribed or doses are variable.

Identifying the factors associated with poor concordance is vital because in doing so those responsible for prescribing and evaluating drug therapy can address the underlying cause and positively influence compliance. A brief examination of these factors shows that individuals who unintentionally fail to take medication as prescribed require different approaches to those failing to take it intentionally. For clinicians working with people with dementia the task may be twofold: to address factors related to intentional nonconcordance and to address those factors associated with unintentional nonconcordance. The main factors associated with unintentional nonconcordance with prescribed medication are highlighted below together with approaches that clinicians can apply to overcome them.

Evidence for Practice

Unintentional Nonconcordance with Prescribed Medication

Underlying cause	Outcome	Clinical approaches
Poor eyesight	Instructions are misinterpreted and medication is not taken or taken inappropriately	Ensure written information is provided in a form the individual can interpret
Verbal instructions are misunderstood	The medication is not taken appropriately	Checking and ensuring the individual's understanding should be part of the consultation process
Poor dexterity	Medication is not taken as the individual cannot open the container	Ensure medication is provided in containers that the individual can manipulate – a physical assessment may be required
Instructions are provided in a language the individual cannot interpret	The medication is not taken or taken inappropriately	Ensure instructions are provided in the individual's first language
Difficulty remembering	Medication is forgotten, taken erratically or too much is taken	Work with the individual to develop the most appropriate method to aid their memory. This may involve trying various approaches like visual or verbal prompt, linking tablet taking to other lifestyle habits, enlisting the help of family or others to prompt, use aids such as a dosset box or blister packs
Polypharmacy	Increased risk of confusion over when and how to take medications	Rationalise numbers and times of medication to a minimum and consult with the individual to develop approaches to ensure that the regime can be managed by the individual. This may include verbal and visual prompts or enlisting the help of others

Overcoming the difficulties that intentional nonconcordance creates can be achieved by increasing the level of consultation prior to the prescription of drug treatments and by monitoring concordance and having an ongoing dialogue with the individual about their experience of using the medication prescribed. There is a requirement that any presumption that individuals with dementia cannot be involved in such consultation does not prevent clinicians from attempting consultation. The aspects to consider in consultation with individuals about their drug treatments which will support concordance are outlined below.

Evidence for Practice

Consultation Aimed at Promoting Concordance Will Include Discussion of the Following

What the medication is for

The benefits and intended outcomes of taking the treatment

Alternatives to the proposed treatment and rationale for why the proposed treatment is preferred

Potential outcome of refusing the treatment

How long the treatment will take to work

How long the treatment is likely to be needed

What the side effects might be and what to do about them

The importance of taking the medicine regularly in the prescribed form in order for it to work properly

The risks associated with stopping the medication suddenly

What to do if a dose is missed or too much is taken

Who to contact and how to contact them if the individual requires information or help with the treatment or treatment effects

Individual concerns

Any potential difficulties the individual may experience in adhering to their prescription and how they may be overcome

How and when the treatment will be monitored and reviewed

The individual's understanding of points discussed

Consent

Ascertaining consent to treatment is a key part of the consultation process and should be established prior to commencement of treatment. Consent to or refusal of treatment in people who retain the ability to decide for themselves is fairly straightforward, but for those people with dementia who are unable to make an informed decision two particularly risky situations can be identified. The first occurs in situations where the individual takes medication because it is offered, with no understanding of what it is or why they are taking it. The second situation is where the individual refuses medication with no understanding of the need for or benefit of the medication. The individual with dementia is likely to be vulnerable and at risk in either situation. It would be very naïve to presume that all medication prescribed for people with dementia will be beneficial. Medication, particularly medication used to control excess behaviour, is not always in the best interest of the individual taking it. The use of medication in this way is discussed further in the next section, but the intricacies of ensuring the individual with dementia has their best interests protected, although of growing interest to the researchers, has yet to produce anything like the level of guidance required to secure the rights of people with dementia.

One aspect impacting on the effectiveness or otherwise of prescribed medication in relation to older adults that can clearly be managed better by clinicians is the routine practice of issuing medication on repeat prescription. Issuing through repeat prescription reduces the opportunity for the person prescribing to monitor the effects and the continued need for the treatment with the person being treated. Repeat prescribing may also increase the risk of errors in prescription and the ability of the individual prescribing to ensure the quantities issued are appropriate for the intended duration of treatment.

It is only by seeing and speaking to an individual that the success or otherwise of a treatment can be evaluated and decisions made about the continued need for each prescribed drug. It is only by speaking to the individual and/or those close to them that it can be discerned that medication prescribed is actually being taken as prescribed and that any difficulties with concordance can be identified and tackled. While the solution may seem as simple as demanding that those prescribing medication, primarily doctors, see the person receiving treatment more often, in reality in terms of time this is difficult to achieve. The Department of Health (2001b) calls for policies and checks to be put in place to ensure that the difficulties identified in issuing medication through repeat prescriptions are addressed. There is a role also for those other than the individual prescribing to observe, discuss and monitor the outcomes of medication and concordance with the person receiving treatment and their carers and to communicate any concerns to the person prescribing in order that the prescription is appropriate to individual need.

Polypharmacy is the term given to the use of multiple medications in an individual's treatment. Polypharmacy is usually a feature where an individual has several coexisting medical conditions, each requiring a pharmaceutical approach. In the care of those over 65 polypharmacy is often viewed as unavoidable as an attempt to manage co-morbidity. However, polypharmacy creates additional difficulties, including the manner in which different drugs interact, the individual's ability to manage complex drug regimes and possible additional side effects, as well as the fact that often different drugs are prescribed by different medical specialists who have little opportunity to communicate with one another concerning the aims of their treatment and how it may impact on what the other specialist is trying to achieve.

In terms of polypharmacy the difficulties created by a requirement to treat individuals who have coexisting illnesses are further complicated in individuals where one of the coexisting conditions is dementia. Here the requirement is to treat both physical ill-health and mental ill-health, which may necessitate the use of an array of drugs aimed at alleviating physical ailments together with antidementia medication. Yet a further layer of complexity may be added where the individual is identified as having psychiatric symptoms, such as hallucinations or paranoia, or where the person presents with so-called challenging behaviours which are traditionally treated with psychotropic preparations. Those prescribing medication may include the psychiatrist, general practitioner and one or more medical specialist, each concentrating on the aims of their particular approach with potentially limited appreciation or understanding of the implications of their approach in terms of what other treatment the individual is receiving. This may further be compounded as traditionally channels of communication between specialists are poor and the person with the fewest specialist skills, the general practitioner, is frequently expected to coordinate the various treatments prescribed. For individuals with dementia the ability to comprehend and comply with a medication regime involving multiple preparations to be taken at various times and in various doses and to interpret changes in themselves as the result of any of the preparations taken makes concordance complicated and monitoring and evaluating outcomes (including side effects) difficult. However difficult the task, the onus remains on the care team to make every effort to ensure that what is prescribed is appropriate to individual need, that the individual has the opportunity to achieve concordance in managing their medicines in order to benefit, that what is prescribed is regularly reviewed for continued appropriateness and that their physical safety and human rights are given apposite and serious consideration.

GENERAL PRINCIPLES OF DRUG TREATMENT IN DEMENTIA CARE

The guiding principle of any approach to care should always be that the approach will benefit the individual and be safe to apply. In dementia care and in respect of drug treatments this guiding principle should be no different. The approach to prescribing and managing medication for people with dementia must address the needs of the individual and specifically how the treatment can be expected to improve what can be improved upon, can control symptoms adversely affecting quality of life and importantly show that the treatment will not result in harm caused by adverse effects, drug interaction or unintentional nonconcordance. The most widely used definition, according to Jackson *et al.* (2003) of what constitutes an appropriate approach in relation to prescription of medication is a risk–benefit approach (defined by the RAND Corporation) where 'the expected health benefit exceeds the expected negative consequences by a sufficiently wide margin that it is worth providing'. By addressing a series of questions, outlined below, clinicians may be able to ensure appropriateness in prescribing.

DO WE NEED TO TREAT WITH MEDICATION?

Although dementia is a progressive syndrome and an individual's needs will change over time, some changes in behaviour and need are to be expected and it should not be a foregone conclusion that a change in need necessitates a change in the care approach. Prior to any decision to treat with drugs, a process of assessment should be undertaken to determine the nature of the symptom or behaviour causing concern. This assessment should include an appraisal of medication the individual is already taking. The aim of this is twofold: to consider whether what the individual is already taking could be contributing to their problems and to ensure clinicians are not misinterpreting an adverse drug reaction as a symptom of ill-health. From the perspective of the individual's current medication regime, stopping what can be stopped, reducing what can be reduced and ensuring times and doses of remaining medications are rationalised so that they can be managed by the individual will be helpful, and indeed may resolve the problem. An important element of the assessment is to give serious consideration to other approaches to managing the symptom or behaviour, for example a psychological or psychosocial approach. Such approaches are likely to be less intrusive and without the potential side effects and adverse events associated with drug treatments. Having undertaken an assessment and ruled out other possible methods of approach it may become evident that drug treatment is identified as the most appropriate response.

WHAT TREATMENT IS APPROPRIATE?

Establishing the appropriate drug for the individual will involve describing the symptom to be treated, consideration of the treatments available, including their efficacy and safety, and consideration of individual factors such as age, other conditions being treated, potential drug interactions and adverse events. Other factors effecting the choice of treatment are those likely to improve the chances of concordance. In this manner the rationale for using a particular medication can be established.

WHAT ARE THE AGREED GOALS OF TREATMENT?

No course of treatment should be undertaken without a clear rationale for the use of that treatment. An initial assessment undertaken correctly should identify the symptoms or behaviour that clinicians are seeking to influence; from there it should be relatively easy to describe what improvement is anticipated and how that improvement would be manifest in the individual's behaviour or presentation. Clarifying the goals of therapy, including clear agreement on the desired outcomes in terms of symptoms and behaviour, will enable clinicians not only to measure the effects of treatment but also to have discussions with the individual which will promote concordance.

IS TREATMENT IN THE BEST INTERESTS OF THE INDIVIDUAL?

In those clients with dementia who retain capacity the onus is on clinicians to provide relevant information in an accessible manner in order that the individual can make a decision about whether or not they will take the medication. As discussed above, there are two situations where people with dementia are particularly vulnerable: where they accept treatment without understanding the purpose or possible side effects and where they refuse treatment and potentially deny themselves the benefit of that treatment. Involving care team members, the individual (where possible) and carers or advocates in discussion about the benefits and risks of the proposed treatment and setting out clear goals in order that efficacy can be evaluated during treatment should contribute to ensuring a decision to treat is taken in the individual's best interest. While such actions may help safeguard the incapacitated client who assents to treatment it is unlikely to ensure that an incapacitated person who dissents will take the medication. In this circumstance there are actions that the care team can attempt in order to encourage assent. For example, consider whether there is something about the form of the medication that the individual may find objectionable or difficult to cope with, the taste, texture or size of a tablet. Providing the medication in a different form such as a syrup or two small tablets instead of a large one may overcome dissent. Consider also whether there are circumstances where the individual does accept medication and whether these circumstances could be replicated on a regular basis – perhaps one person is more successful than others for example. Covert administration of medicine, while legally permissible, may compromise the relationship between the person with dementia and carers, engendering suspicion not only of food or drink (as taste is altered by added medication) but of other actions as well. Thus seeking person centred approaches to concordance with medication, though time consuming, is always more desirable. Treloar *et al.* (2001) suggest that where medication is given covertly the doctor, nurse, pharmacist, relative or advocate should be involved in discussions and a record made of decisions reached.

CAN CONCORDANCE BE ACHIEVED?

Of course having established that incorporating a new drug into the individual's care is likely to be beneficial, there is still the question of concordance. Will the individual take the medication and do so in a way that is safe and optimises the benefits of the drug? As we have seen, consent is only one part of concordance, and for people with dementia difficulties with memory and judgement may certainly contribute to unintentional nonconcordance and raise risks, not only in terms of missed benefits but also of adverse events including overdose. The medication may not be taken at all or may be taken sporadically, it may be taken too frequently and risks may be further increased where more than one medication or dose per day is involved. Adverse effects or side effects of the medication may not be recognised as related to medication and the person may not realise that reporting these effects is important. Some strategies to overcome these problems are suggested in the Evidence for Practice table on Unintentional nonconcordance, given earlier in the chapter. However, it is only by working with the individual that a full assessment of the issues they face in reaping the benefits and avoiding the risks can be made.

HOW WILL THE TREATMENT BE MANAGED?

At the outset of treatment a plan to manage the process of treatment should be discussed. Several roles are required to be undertaken: monitoring for side effects, adverse responses and concordance, taking responsibility for titrating dose and deciding when the treatment is complete or not bringing the anticipated benefit. This plan should ideally involve members of the clinical team, the person receiving treatment and those close to them.

In common with other people, people with dementia can undoubtedly benefit from treatment with drugs. Similarly, they can be at risk of adverse events and unwanted side effects. The problems dementia brings in terms of raising risks of unintentional nonconcordance and age related complications (for those over 65) means that a high level of support is likely to be required to ensure benefits are achieved. An approach that involves all members of the care team, the person themselves (as far as is possible), carers and advocates at all stages of the treatment is appropriate. Such an approach should ensure that the relevant questions are addressed in relation to the individual, that the need for treatment is agreed, the person's rights are protected, the benefits of the treatment outweigh potential negative effects and the course of treatment is evaluated in order that the treatment ceases at the appropriate point.

Evidence for Practice

The Principles of Drug Treatment in Dementia

The guiding principle of drug treatment in dementia care is that treatment is beneficial, safe and in the individual's best interests

A full assessment should be undertaken to ensure drug treatment is the most appropriate course of action

The available treatments should be considered in relation to efficacy and suitability for the individual

The goals of treatment should be agreed and measurable

A person centred approach may overcome dissent to treatment and is more desirable than covert administration of medication

A planned approach involving clinicians, the person treated and their family/advocate at all stages of treatment is appropriate

THE USE OF ANTIPSYCHOTIC MEDICATION IN DEMENTIA CARE

Antipsychotic medications are those drugs developed to treat psychosis in adults generally under 65 years with mental ill-health, including schizophrenia, psychotic illness and bipolar disorder. The drugs of choice include both typical antipsychotic preparations, for example chlorpromazine, promazine and thioridazine and atypical antipsychotic preparations such as olanzapine, quetiapine and risperidone. These medications have traditionally been the first line of treatment for behavioural and psychological symptoms of dementia (BPSD). The high susceptibility of older adults to the side effects of typical antipsychotics, particularly movement disorder such as Parkinsonism, have led to a reliance in more recent years on the newer atypical antipsychotic medications. When we consider that anywhere between 60 and 80 % of people with dementia will experience BPSD throughout the course of their dementia we can see that managing these symptoms effectively is very important.

In Chapter 6 we saw that these symptoms are manifest most frequently in what is commonly referred to as 'challenging behaviour' and are attributed to people with dementia who behave in ways carers find upsetting, difficult to manage, annoying and sometimes physically threatening. Such behaviour includes aggression, constant walking, shouting, verbal repetition or repetitive questioning, actions that are repetitive, disturbed sleeping, food refusal, inappropriate sexual behaviour and incontinence. Despite a growing awareness and some support from the evidence base that psychosocial approaches represent best practice in the management of behavioural and psychological symptoms of dementia, there is still an overreliance on psychotropic medication. Like many aspects of the changing dementia care specialism the evidence for the benefit of psychosocial approaches over the use of psychotropic drugs has yet to infiltrate or influence practice on a wide scale.

The continued widespread use of antipsychotic drug preparations in dementia care is even more difficult to understand when a review of the evidence reveals that not only are the vast majority of these drugs not licensed for use in treatment of dementia symptoms but they are associated with an increased risk of cerebrovascular events, produce only minimum benefit and hasten cognitive decline.

That an increased risk of cerebrovascular adverse events is associated with the use of atypical antipsychotic drugs was uncovered by manufacturers' studies, which were initially designed to try and establish approval for the use of risperidone and olanzapine to control psychotic features of dementia. Subsequent studies led the UK Committee on Safety of Medicines (2004) to issue a warning of the dangers associated with olanzapine and risperidone and to recommend that these drugs should not be initiated with older adults with dementia due to a threefold increase in stroke risk and a twofold risk in mortality.

A further review in 2006 by Ballard and Waite found that while there is evidence that risperidone and olanzapine reduce aggression and risperidone reduces psychosis in dementia, both increase the risk of cerebrovascular events and extrapyramidal side effects. The conclusion was that 'Despite the modest efficacy, the significant increase in adverse events confirms that neither risperidone nor olanzapine should be used routinely to treat dementia patients with aggression or psychosis unless there is marked risk or severe distress.' While such evidence may lead to reliance on atypical antipsychotic medication other than olanzapine and risperidone the risks are not necessarily lower; it may well be that once controlled trials of other preparations (not yet conducted) are completed similar findings will be evident. This evidence may also lead to a return to the use of typical antipsychotics, although Wang *et al.* (2005) caution that if their findings are confirmed these preparations are 'at least as likely as atypical antipsychotic agents to increase the risk of death among elderly persons and that conventional drugs should not be used to replace atypical agents'.

A further concern in relation to the use of antipsychotic medication in dementia care is the potential to hasten cognitive decline. McShane *et al.* (1997) found that the rate of cognitive decline in subjects taking antipsychotics was twice that in those not taking them and that the commencement of treatment was associated with an increase in the rate of decline. A study by Ballard *et al.* (2005) concluded that another of the atypical antipsychotic preparations, quetiapine, as well as being ineffective as a treatment for agitation in people with dementia is associated with greater cognitive decline. If there are approaches to managing BPSD that do not involve the administration of psychotropic medication, if there is mounting evidence of an increased risk to physical health when using antipsychotic medication with people who have dementia, together with evidence that negative cognitive outcomes are associated with using these drugs, and if there is no compelling evidence for their effectiveness, why does practice routinely continue to rely on these drugs?

The answer may lie in several areas. As highlighted in the Royal College of Psychiatrists (RCP) Faculty in the Psychiatry of Old Age prescribing update (2004), the evidence for nonpharmacological approaches to the management of BPSD is not strong enough for any one intervention to be justified as a direct alternative to antipsychotic medication, which may lead clinicians to persist with traditional treatments. Expediency may also account for an overreliance on this medication. The process of developing individualised care can take time. Identifying triggers to behaviour, and finding and implementing approaches that will suit the individual's needs can take weeks. If the behaviour of the individual is severe during this time there may be significant risk to the individual or others where symptoms are uncontrolled. This eventuality may lead clinicians to use antipsychotic medication; indeed, the RCP advice is that in this instance medication should be the first line of response in order to safeguard the individual and others.

However, while it may be safer to use medication to gain rapid control over BPSD to safeguard the person with dementia and those around them, this should not be a replacement for other approaches and should be a short term approach. Where antipsychotic medication is used the RCP counsels that the approach should ensure that treatment targets specific symptoms, that start doses are low and that the treatment time should be limited. This suggests a level of consideration and monitoring that is frequently lacking in many areas where people with dementia with BPSD are currently cared for. A 2006 report issued by the Commission for Social Care Inspection illustrates that 50 % of care homes are not meeting the minimum standards set for managing medication for residents.

We should also consider that our ability to employ environmental or behavioural approaches may be compromised by organisational issues such as low staffing levels, poor training for staff and a reliance on transient staff, all of which mean that recourse to antipsychotic medication may be preferable to the skilled, time consuming and expensive task of establishing and maintaining person centred plans of care.

The use of antipsychotic medication in the care of people with dementia is increasingly controversial; concerns over the dangers associated with the drugs are growing. There is also a steady campaign, by the Alzheimer's Society, to raise awareness of the abuse of this medication in nursing and care homes. The overprescription of these drugs is widely acknowledged and has been referred to as the 'chemical cosh'; use of these drugs is frequently a means of subduing individuals with dementia in order that care can be delivered with more speed and less difficulty.

Individuals with dementia are vulnerable when it comes to medication. They are vulnerable to the effects and side effects of drugs and they are vulnerable because in many cases they are unable to make a decision to accept or reject treatment and are reliant on those providing care to take these decisions. Unfortunately, decisions about care approaches are not always made in the best interests of the person receiving treatment. Thus medication may be offered and taken when it is not in the individual's best interests and offered and refused when it is in the individual's best interests. Those providing care are the gatekeepers and the decisions they make and the actions they take will have strong outcomes in terms of quality of life for those in their care. In terms of using antipsychotic drugs we should remember that the evidence shows many of these drugs can increase the risk of cerebrovascular events, have minimum effectiveness and contribute to a hastening of cognitive impairment. Where they are used they should be considered a temporary, emergency approach at a minimum dose to be reduced and ceased as soon as possible – an adjunct to the development of psychosocial and environmental approaches rather than a convenient alternative. One area of research that may yet provide a drug-based approach to the management of BPSD is that into the benefits of acetylcholinesterase inhibitors as a treatment for these symptoms. Overshott and Burns (2005) suggest there is evidence that these drugs, generally the first line of treatment for Alzheimer's disease, can be beneficial in the treatment of agitation, apathy and psychosis in dementia.

Applying the principles underpinning the use of drug treatment in dementia care, as outlined above, may ensure that where these drugs are considered as a treatment for an individual with dementia due consideration is given to relevant issues to provide a clear rationale and plan for the use of such drugs.

Evidence for Practice

The Use of Antipsychotic Medication in Dementia Care

Typical and atypical antipsychotic medications are used, off-license, in dementia care to treat behavioural and psychological symptoms of dementia (BPSD)

Typical antipsychotic preparations have been associated with a high incidence of side effects, particularly movement disorders

The atypical antipsychotics risperidone and olanzapine have been associated with a threefold increase in the risk of stroke and should not be instigated as treatment for BPSD

The evidence for the benefits of some antipsychotic medications is modest

Antipsychotic medication should be one of several approaches used in managing BPSD

There may be an overreliance on these drugs as they are cheaper than psychosocial approaches

Where antipsychotic medications are proposed for use the underpinning principles of drug treatment should be employed

Research indicates that acetylcholinesterase inhibitors may have a role to play in treating BPSD in the future

---

TREATMENTS FOR DEMENTIA

One of the most important changes in the world of dementia care over the past 10 years has been the progress made in developing drugs hailed as a treatment for dementia. As we have seen in Chapter 2, the importance of these developments and accompanying debate in propelling Alzheimer's disease (AD) and dementia to the forefront of the media and public attention has been invaluable. The main medications used to treat dementia are outlined below.

ACETYLCHOLINESTERASE INHIBITORS

Scientists identified in the 1970s that the brains of individuals with AD are deficient in a neurotransmitter called acetylcholine. Acetylcholine is linked to memory performance and is broken down in the brain by acetylcholinesterase. It is this enzyme that the antidementia drugs aim to affect, in order to make more acetylcholine available and increase memory performance. These drugs are also termed cholinesterase inhibitors. The introduction, in 1993, of the first drug approved for the treatment of AD generated hope for those suffering from a disease singularly lacking in hope. This first cholinesterase inhibitor, tacrine, is rarely used today due to side effects and the drugs of choice are now donepezil (Aricept), rivastigmine (Exelon) and galantamine (Reminyl).

The evidence supports that in AD these drugs, when compared with a placebo, have benefits in cognitive function, performance of activities of daily living and the severity of dementia (Birks *et al.* 2000; Birks & Harvey 2003; Loy & Schneider 2004). It is also held that the drugs slow the rate of progression of dementia. The side effects commonly experienced when taking these drugs are gastrointestinal disturbances: nausea, vomiting and diarrhoea. These side effects generally pass over a period of weeks and can be reduced by taking the tablets with food.

In a 2006 review Birks found all three drugs were efficacious in mild to moderate AD, although acting in slightly different ways they were found to be equally effective. Donepezil was found to cause fewest side effects but side effects related to the other drugs could be controlled if the dose was titrated slowly.

Several practice guidelines concur on the following approach to the initiation and management of drug treatments for AD. The treatment is for those diagnosed with AD only, treatment should be initiated by a specialist, early monitoring for compliance and tolerance is necessary, there should be continued evaluation of the effects of the treatment at no less than six-monthly intervals and deterioration in cognition (generally measured as below 12 on the Mini-Mental State Examination) should prompt cessation of treatment. Although licensed in the United Kingdom there has been controversy over their provision under the National Health Service (NHS) since their introduction. These drugs are expensive, approximately £1000 per individual per year; for many this cost is prohibitive. The availability of the drugs under the NHS largely determines an individual's ability to benefit from them.

The availability of cholinesterase inhibitors through the NHS is determined by the recommendations of the National Institute for Health and Clinical Excellence (NICE), the independent organisation responsible for providing national guidance on the treatment of ill-health. In 2001 NICE recommended the use of donepezil, rivastigmine and galatamine for the treatment of mild to moderate AD. However, new draft guidance (2005), while still maintaining that the drugs are an effective and safe treatment, concluded that the drugs were not cost effective and should not be available through the NHS.

On the whole, within a health care service where funds are limited we can understand the need to balance efficacy with cost and ration treatments accordingly. Difficulty arises where you, someone you are close to or the service you are trying to provide is perceived to suffer as a result of the judgement of others that the benefit does not justify the cost and treatment is denied. The strength of the feeling of injustice that those with AD and their carers (formal and informal) brought to bear through campaigning for the availability of cholinesterase inhibitors brought about a hasty change in judgement by NICE. This was achieved not by raising the voice of complaint alone but by highlighting a potential flaw in the approach NICE took in calculating the cost–benefit ratio of the drugs, namely not giving enough considera- tion to the outcomes in terms of quality of life for individuals taking the drugs and their families.

The benefits of cholinesterase inhibitors, campaigners pointed out, should not be calculated purely in terms of scores on cognitive and functioning tests but rather in the quality of life of the individual and those around them. Banerjee *et al.* (2006) point out that relying on assessment of cognition or function as a measure of quality of life is likely to miss important factors concerning life quality. Added to this they highlight the fact that 'Data on the quality of life impacts of dementia are simply not available at present and this makes any assessment of cost effectiveness of dementia treatments, such as that proposed by NICE, highly speculative at the least.' A re-draft was issued for consultation in January 2006 recommending that the drugs should be available for moderate AD. Little explanation as to why it should not be provided for those with mild AD, despite a finding by Birks (2006) that the drugs were efficacious in people with mild AD, was forthcoming. The argument as to the clinical efficacy of these drugs as a treatment for AD seems to have been won but the argument as to their economic efficacy, whether they represent value for money, appears set to rumble on for some time yet.

Although the majority of people who develop dementia will have AD there remains a large proportion of individuals who will not and for whom the argument about the clinical and economic efficacy of cholinesterase inhibitors is mainly academic. There have been studies into the effectiveness of cholinesterase inhibitors for other demen- tia conditions such as Lewy body dementia and future research may broaden the spectrum of those with dementia who may benefit from these drugs. However, there has been some, albeit muted, questioning of the furore about the cholinesterase in- hibitors from within the dementia care specialism, with some commentators pointing out that meeting the costs of cholinesterase inhibitors in reality, being funded from the overall dementia care budget, detracts from funding available for others with dementia.

MEMANTINE

Memantine has been used as a treatment for AD, vascular and mixed dementia in Germany for over 20 years. It is the only drug licensed for use in the treatment of moderate to severe AD in the United Kingdom. It is believed that too much stimulation of nerve cells by a neurotransmitter called glutamate may be respon- sible for the degeneration of brain nerves that happens in AD, vascular dementia or mixed dementia. Once released, glutamate attaches to a receptor on the surface of cells called the *N*-methyl-D-aspartate receptor. It is this receptor that meman- tine blocks thus, it is thought, protecting the nerve cells. The latest consultation draft by NICE recommends against the use of memantine on the grounds of cost effectiveness.

GINKGO BILOBA

Ginkgo biloba is used in other European countries in the treatment of conditions as diverse as confusion, memory disorders, depression and anxiety. It is thought to act as a neuroprotective agent and to increase blood supply to the brain. A review by Birks and Grimley Evans (2002) of trials into the efficacy of Gingko biloba as a treatment for dementia concluded that there is 'promising evidence of improvement in cognition and function associated with Ginkgo' but that more trials were required to quantify treatment effects.

OTHER TREATMENTS

Vascular dementia, accounting for the second highest proportion of those living with dementia, is treated mainly by trying to control risk factors associated with vascular events. This approach is largely health promotion aimed at smoking cessation, diet control and weight loss, as well as treatments to manage blood pressure and cholesterol levels. Other drugs have been used to try and treat dementia, including oestrogen, nonsteroidal anti-inflammatory drugs, selegiline and vitamin E, but clinical trials have not supported their use. Benzodiazepines and hypnotics are also used to promote the control of anxiety and sleep disturbance in dementia care, but in both classes of drugs oversedation is a risk and positive outcomes are debatable. Clinical trials do not support their use.

Evidence for Practice

Treatments for Dementia

The first treatment for Alzheimer's disease, called cholinesterase inhibitors, became available in 1993

These drugs are safe and effective and outcomes include improvement in cognition, functioning and severity of disease in AD

The drugs cost on average £1000 per individual per year and are at present available through the NHS for those diagnosed with moderate dementia

Memantine is the only drug licensed for use in treatment of moderate to severe AD in the United Kingdom, but is not available through the NHS

Ginkgo biloba has also been used as a treatment for dementia, but more studies into its effectiveness have been called for and it is currently not licensed specifically as a treatment for dementia in the United Kingdom

---

CONCLUSION

By and large the content of this book is concerned with building a picture of the context of dementia in today's society and in examining the evidence that has come to light about dementia and the experience of dementia over the past 20 years. This is demanding urgent change in the way dementia is viewed and the way care is practised. This involves consideration of what has long been accepted as traditional care approaches, consultation of the evidence and definition of new practice that incorporates the evidence. Consideration is given here to drug treatment in dementia not only because there have been important developments in drug treatments for Alzheimer's disease but also because this is a neglected area in the general literature about dementia. All too often practitioners see drug treatment as the preserve of medical staff and opportunities for ensuring people who have dementia benefit from drug treatments and avoid the perils of drug misuse are overlooked.

The starting point for pharmacotherapy in dementia care must be in establishing that there is a role for drug treatment, that drug treatment is safe and that the treatment under consideration will benefit the individual. The difficulties identified with managing drug treatments with older adults are likely to be exacerbated in older adults who also have dementia. In order that individuals with dementia can best benefit from prescription drugs the process of prescribing, ensuring and monitoring concordance and evaluating the effects of the drug must be rigorous and involve all clinicians, the person themselves (where possible) and their carer or advocate.

It may be difficult to consult fully with some people with dementia but consultation should always be pursued and the potential for both intentional and nonintentional nonconcordance investigated. Drug treatment is an area where people with dementia are vulnerable, particularly where their capacity to agree to the treatment has been compromised and they are reliant on others to make judgements for them.

Where drug treatment is being considered as an approach to managing behaviour deemed challenging it should be one of the approaches under consideration and generally used only where a trial of other approaches has failed. In a small number of cases, where there is danger to others or the individual themselves, treatment may be a justifiable initial response. It must be remembered that many of the antipsychotic medications used primarily with younger adults with psychotic illness have proved dangerous when used with older adults with dementia.

The progress made in developing drug treatments for dementia, particularly AD, has been fairly dramatic over the past decade and is likely to continue apace. The financial support from the drug companies alone will sustain research into the treatment and cure of dementia. The proportion of the aged population is increasing year on year and with it the numbers of people living with dementia. For the drug companies, finding a treatment and cure for dementia is a lucrative prospect. This is, of course, good news but one wonders what could be achieved if similar levels of financial support were available for investigation into other approaches to care and treatment of dementia. Heller and Heller (2003), in considering the position of drugs in the arena of dementia care, highlight the manner in which the medical model, the pressure from drug companies and a lack of appreciation of the need to fund person centred approaches may lead to continued dominance of medical approaches to the detriment of other approaches, particularly where there is competition for funding. In many respects it may not be useful to see drug treatments and person centred approaches as mutually exclusive, but if the expenditure on developing drug treatments remains disproportionately high, and with the application of drug treatment largely being very much less labour intensive than person centred approaches, there is a danger that the development of opportunities for improving quality of life through person to person approaches will be delayed or even eventually lost.

9 Growing Old and Dying with Dementia

INTRODUCTION

The view of dementia as a progressive syndrome where individuals proceed from one stage to the next and eventually die is somewhat simplistic; individuals rarely fit neatly into one category or progress to the next at any predictable rate. Estimating the length of time someone will live with dementia is difficult and dependent on variable factors, including the type of dementia, coexisting conditions, place of care and quality of care. Studies into survival time following the onset of dementia generally report a survival time of between 3 and 9 years, although there is no doubt that some individuals live upwards of 20 years with dementia and yet others survive only months following onset. Some studies (Knopman *et al.* 2003; Fitzpatrick *et al.* 2005) found a lower median survival time in vascular dementia than Alzheimer's disease. Policy makers have an interest in establishing how long people will live with dementia as it enables estimates concerning the amount of care likely to be required to be made and budgets to be planned.

However, arguably of more interest to us, as carers, is how we can contribute to good quality of life for the individual at any stage of their illness. This may be particularly important where the individual is experiencing advanced dementia and where global impairment compromises the ability in virtually all areas of cognition and functioning and the individual is dependent on others to sustain life and life quality. At this point physical and mental health problems are likely to be complex and multiple and further complicated by ethical and legal issues. Individuals will live with advanced dementia on average for 18 months to 2 years, although some may survive up to 10 years. The vulnerability of individuals at this stage of living with and dying with dementia is extremely high and the standard of care and the monitoring of that care must be equally high. Unfortunately this is not always or, perhaps, even often the case.

This chapter looks at living and dying with advanced dementia. The chapter begins with a review of the signs and symptoms of advanced dementia. The subject of abuse is examined: the types of abuse individuals may be vulnerable to, how this abuse is manifest and the responsibilities, particularly of professional carers, to ensure people with dementia are protected from abuse. There is discussion also of advance statements and directives, and how dialogue between clinicians and individuals can facilitate both quality of life and decision making in severe dementia. The chapter also considers how we are currently meeting the needs of those dying with dementia and how taking a palliative approach to the care of people living and dying with dementia can contribute to person centred care.

ADVANCED DEMENTIA

The collection of symptoms that comprise dementia are progressive from minor to severe as the disease advances. While minor symptoms of early stage dementia disrupt accustomed routines, create daily difficulties and bring distressing emotional challenges for both the carer and the person with the syndrome, it is during the advanced stage that the full impact of dementia is realised. It is at this stage that all that has become difficult throughout the experience of dementia largely becomes impossible. The level of disability and need that severe dementia creates in an individual means that in an ideal care situation the expertise of multiple professionals is desirable. In the United Kingdom at present this almost inevitably means that the individual living with severe dementia will do so in an institutional setting.

Judgement, planning and sequencing skills are so damaged by this stage of dementia that the person will be unable to recognise or respond to even their basic daily needs for cleansing, clothing, comfort and nutrition. Dysphasia and aphasia are features and compromise expressive communication and the individual's ability to receive and decipher the communication of others is also significantly impaired. Gross motor coordination becomes impaired and may impact on mobility, self-care and eating and drinking activities. In the final throes of the disease contracture of limbs is common. Incontinence is a feature of advanced dementia and dysphagia means that ensuring comfortable and adequate nutrition and fluids is difficult.

Socially the individual may become completely isolated and withdrawn as their ability to interact or seek social contact is disabled and the opportunity and specialist support may not be forthcoming to sustain emotional well-being or a sense of self. By this stage the person is unlikely to be able to demonstrate that they recognise those close to them. This can be particularly upsetting for spouse and family members. Individuals may behave in ways termed challenging, acting in an aggressive manner, shouting, walking continuously or incessantly repeating movements or actions in an apparently meaningless way. There are real risks, as we have seen, of this behaviour being interpreted as symptomatic of dementia and resulting in inappropriate use of medication. The consequences of this global deterioration for the individual are numerous and the risk of further physical health complications, for example malnutrition, pressure sores, repeat and severe infections, is high, particularly as the individual is unable to recognise that something is wrong or to express discomfort in ways that are easy to comprehend.

Although not recognised as a terminal disease, once an individual develops dementia they will have it until they die. Unlike many other chronic diseases the point of death is difficult to predict. For those of us who do not have dementia, observing the vulnerability of an individual with this level of need and disability, together with the isolation that communication barriers create, means that the thought of having to live with advanced dementia is, at the very least, a frightening prospect.

However, other care specialisms have something to teach those of us caring for people with advanced dementia. For example, those specialising in care of people with cancer have expertly demonstrated that the individual faced with the prospect of an unpleasant and drawn-out death can be enabled to live their life to as full an extent as possible within the strictures the disease imposes, with an acceptable degree of life quality, in consultation with care providers, and to face death with dignity and in the knowledge that those close to them will be supported during bereavement. This is what we should be striving towards in dementia care: to enable individuals living and dying with severe dementia to do so with dignity, in comfort, in the company of those who are important to them, in familiar surroundings, free from pain and in the manner they have negotiated with those delivering the care that they require. A key component to this process will be the consultation between the person with dementia and carers. As we have seen throughout this book, supporting any consultation presents an immense challenge and it is only through taking on this challenge and finding ways to meet it that the quality of care people with dementia receive is likely to develop to an expert level that is universally available.

VULNERABILITY AND ABUSE OF PERSONS WITH ADVANCED DEMENTIA

The cognitive and functional impact of dementia means that individuals become increasingly dependent on others to meet their needs, from the most basic of survival needs such as food, shelter and warmth to the psychosocial needs for communication, occupation and relationship. There are two primary considerations: firstly, these needs are met and, secondly, they are met in a way that respects the individual's accustomed standards and desires. It would be comforting to believe that both these considerations are addressed on a daily basis for people living with advanced dementia but we know from media reports and indeed frequently from our own clinical experience that there is much yet to be done.

For people living with advanced dementia this increasing level of dependence means that their vulnerability to abuse is extremely high. The stark truth is that people with dementia, in particular people with severe dementia, are at high risk of being abused, and indeed are being abused as I write this and as you read it, in their own homes, in nursing homes, in residential homes and in hospitals. They are abused by relatives, friends, neighbours, nurses, doctors, carers, strangers and loved ones. They are at risk of being abused wherever they are and by whomever they have contact with. The risk of abuse and the actuality of abuse are facts that carers, particularly professional carers, need to be aware of and alert to in their daily practice, in order that they can contribute to the protection of those in their care.

The British Geriatric Society (2005) defines abuse of older adults as 'a single or repeated act or lack of appropriate action occurring within any relationship where there is an expectation of trust which causes harm or distress to an older person'. The British Geriatric Society identifies people with dementia as more commonly subject to abuse than other sectors of the older adult community. It is estimated that half a million older people suffer abuse in the United Kingdom. The likelihood is that the real figure is significantly higher as many cases go unreported, due to fear, inability to communicate, lack of opportunity and perhaps most alarmingly because reports by people with dementia are not given credence. Abuse can take several forms: physical, sexual, financial and emotional abuse, abuse through neglect and discrimination.

Physical abuse is the use of physical force against an individual that inflicts pain, injury and suffering. Examples of physical abuse include hitting, slapping, pinching, restraint, rough handling, overuse or underuse of medication and force feeding. The signs of physical abuse may be easier to interpret than other types of abuse as the results are often visible in the form of bruising, broken bones and oversedation. However, such signs may be hidden and other indicators are sudden changes in the behaviour of the person with dementia, shrinking from the touch of others and self-reporting, although first hand accounts by the individual are in danger of being interpreted as the result of dementia rather than a factual account by the individual of their circumstances. Vague or inconsistent accounts by others of how injuries were sustained may also indicate a case of abuse.

Sexual abuse may be defined as any sexual contact that is nonconsensual. For individuals with advanced dementia where capacity has been lost any sexual contact must be considered to constitute abuse. Examples of sexual abuse are intimate touching, fondling, forced sexual acts, situations where the person is unnecessarily naked, sexual teasing or conversation and forced viewing of pornography. The signs of such abuse include bruising on the thighs or genitals, anal or genital bleeding and sexually transmitted infections. As with most instances of abuse, a change in usual behaviour and self-reporting are signs of abuse, but there is a real danger that both are interpreted as symptomatic of dementia and individuals remain at risk.

Financial abuse is the illegal or unauthorised use of an individual's money, assets or property. It may involve stealing money or property, selling assets, making the individual sign cheques or legal papers granting another right over property or assets, overcharging for services and misuse of credit cards. Signs that financial abuse is happening may comprise money or other assets disappearing, observation of others making the person sign papers or cheques and inflated bills. The individual may also behave other than usual and may express concern about their money or belongings. The perpetrator of this abuse may be reluctant to discuss financial affairs with others or to disclose financial information when required.

Emotional or psychological abuse is behaviour or communication on the part of others that leaves the individual distressed, frightened, intimidated or isolated. Such behaviour includes verbal threats, humiliation, harassment and intimidation. Kitwood (1997), when describing what he termed a 'malignant social psychology', which can surround people with dementia, gives clear examples of the type of behaviour on the part of carers that constitutes emotional abuse. Although any type of abuse may be part of a care culture in institutional settings this type of abuse is arguably the most pervasive. Obviously cruel in nature, such behaviour is deemed permissible on the (false) basis that the individual does not understand what is being said. The hope is that once uninformed carers practising this type of abuse are educated to understand the impact of their behaviour positive change through education can be enabled. The impact of emotional abuse on the quality of life of the individual with advanced dementia is significant and can generate anxiety, distress and withdrawal, all of which may be evident in the person's behaviour. Where such a culture persists it may be relatively easy for outsiders to observe the behaviour of the perpetrator, which is likely to be domineering, dictatorial, bullying and taunting in nature. Although the perpetrators may have enough insight to realise that hiding such behaviour is in their best interests, it may only be when a new member of staff arrives that the potential for recognition of the abusive situation arises.

Abuse by neglect may be physical or emotional. Physical neglect is the nonprovision or inappropriate provision of basic physical requirements such as food, fluids, heat, clothing, hygiene, adequate opportunity to use the toilet, lack of assistance to mobilise and lack of attention to health needs. Emotional neglect may include ignoring requests for help, ignoring moans or signs of distress, leaving the person with dementia alone for prolonged periods, restriction of visitors or contact with the outside world and lack of opportunity to be occupied or engaged in relationships that offer affection. Again one of the signs of neglect may be that the person reports it; other signs include dehydration, poor living conditions with poor heating supply or inadequate facilities to meet basic needs, dishevelled or dirty appearance, pressure sores and social withdrawal or behaviour termed challenging on the part of the victim of the abuse.

Discriminatory abuse is harmful behaviour targeted at an individual on the basis of their race, sexuality, gender, age, disability or cultural or religious beliefs. It involves name calling, verbal abuse, isolating the individual from activity or events in their environment, denying culturally appropriate diet or attendance to religious or culturally important rituals. Discriminatory abuse may result in other types of abuse. Signs include evidence that the individual is not as well cared for as others in the care environment, withdrawal by the individual from social contact and depression. For ease of reference types, examples and signs of abuse are illustrated in the table at the end of this section.

The incidence of abuse may be a one-off outburst or systematic, planned and sustained. Some causes of abuse or neglect are unintentional and result from lack of awareness, training or knowledge of the consequences of actions or how to overcome problems. Abuse may result from carer stress, isolation or from the carer's own mental or physical health difficulties.

The Commission for Health Improvement (2003) identifies the known factors for abuse in institutional settings as a poor and institutionalised environment, poor clinical supervision, a closed and inward looking culture, low staffing levels with high use of agency or bank staff, poor staff development and poor management.

Other causes of abuse lie in family relationships, or patterns of behaviour within families. There can also be no doubt that some people abuse, threaten or neglect people with dementia simply because they have the opportunity and they believe they can get away with it, as the likelihood of the subject of the abuse being able to report it or to have such a report believed is low.

The consequences of abuse for people with dementia include an exacerbation of dementia and dependence, dehydration and malnutrition, loss of assets, depression, loss of contact with the social world, loss of esteem and dignity, physical injury and even death. The job of identifying and tackling abuse of its most vulnerable members is obviously the responsibility of society as a whole, but as the British Geriatric Society (2005) recognises the level and nature of the contact those who provide specialist services to older adults have places them in a key position to identify, report and manage abuse. This will obviously require that those with this level of contact have access to training and the organisational structures that will facilitate their ability to do so effectively. The Department of Health and Home Office (2000) and the Department of Health (2004) seek to direct those across organisations to develop multiagency codes of practice in reducing elder abuse and this will undoubtedly help.

Those working to professional codes of practice are also obligated through these codes to protect the interests of those they are professionally responsible for. This will include the code of practice accompanying the planned Mental Capacity Act due to be implemented in 2007. This act will, for the first time, see bad treatment of someone who lacks capacity defined as a criminal offence, which will hopefully aid the fight to stamp out abuse of people with dementia.

At ground level one of the major ways forward is for each individual who recognises the behaviour of others as a form of abuse or suspects abuse is occurring to step forward and 'blow the whistle'. This is particularly important in 24-hour care settings and is particularly difficult due to the pressure individuals feel working in these settings where the demand to conform is great and an incentive to inform is poor.

As we have seen throughout this book, developing expertise in dementia care is extremely challenging, but is driven by evidence, by compassion and by a desire to deliver care that is person centred. The protection of vulnerable people with dementia from abuse is fundamental to the theory of our practice and must be central to implementation of our practice.

Evidence for Practice

Types of Abuse

Type of abuse	Examples of abuse	Signs of abuse
Physical	Punching, striking, pinching, pushing, rough handling, slapping, restraint, overuse or underuse of medication	Bruising, fractures, oversedation, self-report, changes in behaviour, shrinking away at the approach or touch of others, inconsistent or unbelievable accounts by others as to how an injury was sustained
Sexual	Intimate touching, fondling, forced sexual acts, situations where the	Bruising on the thighs or genitals, anal or genital bleeding and sexually

(*Continued*)

	person is unnecessarily naked, sexual teasing or conversation and forced viewing of pornography	transmitted infections, self-report, change in behaviour
Financial	Theft of money or property, sale of assets, making the individual sign cheques or legal papers granting another right over property or assets, overcharging for services, misuse of credit cards	Money or other assets disappearing, observation of others making the person sign papers or cheques, inflated bills, reluctance on the part of those controlling assets to discuss their use, concern expressed by the person with dementia
Emotional or psychological	Use of behaviour or communication that belittles, humiliates, dominates, threatens, bullies, taunts or isolates	Person with dementia is withdrawn, anxious, depressed, distressed, self-reports
Physical neglect	Inappropriate provision of food, fluids, heat, clothing, hygiene, inadequate opportunity to use the toilet, lack of assistance to mobilise, lack of attention to health needs	Dehydration and malnutrition, poor living conditions, inadequate facilities to meet basic needs, dishevelled or dirty appearance, pressure sores, repeat infections, severe infection that could have been treated sooner, self-report
Emotional neglect	Requests for help are ignored, expressions of distress are ignored, the person is left alone for prolonged periods, visitors and contact with the outside world are restricted, opportunity to be occupied or engaged in relationships is denied	Self-report, withdrawal, depression, self-stimulation including rocking, repetitive actions, shouting

(*Continued*)

Discriminatory	Name calling, verbal abuse, isolating the individual from activity or events in their environment, denying culturally appropriate diet or attendance to religious or culturally important rituals, any other type of abuse	Signs that the individual is not as well cared for as others in the same environment, withdrawal by the individual from social contact and depression, self-report

CONSULTING ON THE FUTURE

One of the dilemmas for clinicians when an individual is diagnosed with early stage dementia is how much to tell the individual and those close to them about the trajectory of the disease and what they can expect to happen to them. There are many aspects to this dilemma; the discomfiture of the clinician in having to detail such devastating information, the concern that the person may attempt suicide if they are given such information, pressure from the family not to provide the information and of course the fact that not every individual will experience all the features or the progression to the advanced stage of dementia. However, for those who do live long enough with dementia the consequences of not preparing them or their loved ones for the event of living with severe dementia can directly impact on the quality of life and the quality of death of the person and those close to them.

Inevitably, as with any illness or disease process, decisions will have to be made about the type of medical and care interventions the person receives. For people with dementia, because their capacity to make decisions and express choices is eroded as the disease advances, a staged approach to obtaining subjective wishes as situations arise is not possible. The current approach in practice, once the person is deemed to have lost the capacity to make decisions for themselves, largely involves discussions between the clinical care team and family aimed at trying to determine what the person would have wanted could they have been involved in the decision making process. What this approach attempts to do is to harness what those who were close to the individual prior to their having dementia know about the individual's life values in order to estimate what their opinion on the current situation might be. While such an approach tries to include the opinion of the individual receiving care by proxy it is likely to prove flawed. A study undertaken by Vig *et al.* (2002) found that an individual's current values are not easily translated into end of life preferences. For example, it might be predicted that individuals with close family relationships would want family members present at the time of death, but Vig *et al.* found that this was not the case and for other reasons individuals in close family relationships did not want loved ones present at the time of death. While the Vig *et al.* study was relatively small the implications are huge; we should not extrapolate what we think the person would want from what we know of their past expressed preferences. Relying too much on the views of family or those close to the individual presents other difficulties. Forbes *et al.* (2000) describe how the unresolved needs of family members, together with a lack of information and emotional support, meant they were unprepared for making treatment decisions. If we are going to place family members in the position of influencing decision making for individuals with advanced dementia then we must also take responsibility for ensuring they are supported both emotionally and with regard to the quality and quantity of information they receive, in order to ensure that their decisions are informed by facts that are relevant rather than carried on pure emotion based on their relationship with the person who must experience the outcome of the decision.

An alternative to relying on family or those close to the person when decisions are required to be made is to consult with the individual while they still have capacity. This approach, seen as improving consultation and planning for the future and aimed at extending the autonomy of the individual past the time when they have the capacity to make decisions, is to use an advance statement or an advance directive.

An advance statement is a declaration of the individual's wishes and opinions, a way to state preferences and specify the forms of medical treatment that would or would not be acceptable should the individual at some point in the future be unable to be involved in discussions or make an informed choice about the treatment. An advance statement can include information on life values, religious or spiritual beliefs that would inform any decision making and indeed care processes on an ongoing basis. The individual can also use an advance statement to nominate someone they would like to be consulted on their behalf at a time when a decision is required. Advance statements are not legally binding.

An advance directive allows the individual to refuse some or all forms of medical treatment in certain circumstances. The forms of treatment and the circumstances must be specified and the directive can only be applied to the treatment and in circumstances outlined, and only when the individual no longer retains capacity.

Although there is much talk in the world of dementia care about the desirability of people with dementia completing advance statements and advance directives in order to offer direction for those providing for their future needs, there is little evidence that clinicians are facilitating that process, and it is rare for individuals presently receiving care with severe dementia or dying with dementia to have such a document informing their care. A Debate of the Age Health and Care Study Group (1999) includes being able to issue an advance directive to ensure wishes are respected as one of the 12 principles of a good death and, as Lyness (2004) observes, 'The diagnosis of dementia provides an opportunity (indeed, mandates that we) engage in ongoing end-of-life discussions with the patient and family.' Doing so, he observes, will enable us to elicit values and care preferences that will support a palliative approach to care as the disease progresses. Taking this approach will also give the individual some assurance that when the time comes and they are unable to contribute to major decisions about what happens to them enough information will be available to the carers to ensure that they can act as the individual would want.

Clinicians at the point of diagnosis and those involved in the continued care and support of people with dementia and their families are well placed to instigate and support discussions about living with and dying with dementia and to introduce the idea of advance statements and directives. The issues under discussion are obviously likely to be difficult and emotionally charged, but they are also an opportunity to raise issues with those close to the person with dementia and to relieve some of the onus of decision making by the family at what may be extremely stressful times in the future. The introduction of the Mental Capacity Act early in 2007 should begin to address some of the grey areas in the law in relation to advance decision making and the role of professional carers in supporting those in their care in coming to decisions and recording them in a way that leaves a clear indication of the individual's desires.

Advance statements and directives are certainly gaining in popularity among clinicians, but caution has been expressed by some commentators (Hughes *et al.* 2004) about whether advance directives will be applicable to current circumstances and whether the individual who made the advance directive is the same person as the one now living with severe dementia. For example, a person without dementia or with early stage dementia may decide that the prospect of living with severe dementia offers no quality of life and therefore may make an advance directive refusing a potentially life-extending treatment in the circumstances of them having severe dementia. However, at some point in the future in the reality of their having severe dementia they may demonstrate through their behaviour and communication that they are content and objective assessment may indicate they have a good quality of life. We cannot at that point obtain a decision about their preference for life-extending treatment due to loss of capacity, but must rely on the advance directive. Is it still ethically right to withhold the treatment? Legally we have little choice as an advance directive is legally binding.

Clinicians are faced with simpler but ethically challenging situations on a daily basis. An example from my own practice is the lady with advanced dementia who had practised a religion that restricted the type of fluids taken and who had not taken tea or coffee for many years yet requested tea on a regular basis. Some members of the staff team felt her current expression should be respected and gave her tea, others felt strongly that her lifestyle commitment to her religion should be upheld and did not provide tea. I still do not know which course of action was correct.

In essence the conundrum is this: can we be sure that what an individual says now about what they want in the future in certain circumstances will definitely hold true for that individual once those circumstances are upon them? As Casarett and Karlawish (1999) point out, 'Any form of advance directive is at best an imperfect approximation of a patient's autonomous preferences, never a clear expression of them.'

Advance directives are useful, they can extend the autonomy of individuals who through illness or injury lose capacity, but they are not the panacea they may first appear. People do change, they change as their circumstances change and as they adapt to new circumstances and what once seemed unacceptable becomes acceptable. People with dementia experience arguably more change than most illnesses or diseases impose because it is not only physical circumstances and abilities that alter. However, we should not ignore the capacity of the person experiencing severe dementia to enjoy life and should include this in discussing and planning for the future with people in early stage dementia. Hughes *et al.* (2004) suggest that 'respecting a person's autonomy will require not only attention to past wishes, but also an awareness of the person's current physical, psychological, social and spiritual circumstances'. This leads us back to the way we communicate with people with severe dementia and what we can come to understand about their quality and enjoyment of life from our communication with them, for it is understanding this that will enable appropriate decisions to be made about both care and treatment for that individual.

Evidence for Practice

Advance Statements and Directives

Offer a means by which the autonomy of a person with dementia can be extended beyond a time when they are considered to have lost mental capacity

Involves the person expressing preferences for forms of medical treatments, refusing specified treatments, nominating someone to act on their behalf and providing information on values and spiritual beliefs with the aim of informing future care plans

Can create the opportunity for individuals and those close to them to discuss the future, the situations they may find themselves in and to have support and to support one another in addressing the issues

Can relieve family and others from making important decisions at stressful times in the future

Clinicians involved in disclosing a diagnosis and in follow-up care are well placed to instigate and support these difficult discussions

Clinicians must be abreast of current research in order to enable individuals and those close to them to make informed decisions

The Mental Capacity Act planned to come into force in 2007 should support both professionals and those in their care in providing clear guidelines for reaching and recording advance decisions

Some concern has been raised about whether the individual with early stage dementia is the same person as the one experiencing severe dementia and whether the advance directive is still in the person's best interest

Some commentators suggest an approach that combines information from advance statements and what is observed of the individual's current situation may prove more person centred

CARING FOR PEOPLE DYING WITH DEMENTIA

The way in which people with dementia are cared for as they approach the end of life is influenced by the model of care employed. As we have seen repeatedly throughout this book, dementia care has long been delivered under a model of medical care, based firmly in approaches that seek treatment and cure. As we have also seen, this approach is increasingly being questioned and other approaches aiming to improve quality of life, uphold individual rights and reinforce the individual's self-esteem and their place in the social milieu are now recognised as representing a better way forward. For individuals approaching the end of life with dementia these factors are no less important and the consequences of continuing to deliver care based on the medical model are causing unnecessary suffering.

In practice the application of a medical model of care means that there is frequently no distinction between the care offered to those living with dementia and those dying with dementia. As death approaches for most individuals with a terminal disease the concentration of caring effort revolves around ensuring control of physical and psychological symptoms, promoting comfort, tending to the needs of those close to the person dying and promoting what could be termed a good death. This is possible because the point of death in most disease processes can be predicted with a fair degree of confidence and there can be communication between the carer and cared for almost to the point of death. In dementia care this is very difficult. Estimating survival time even with advanced dementia is not easy, which has led to a tendency not to view dementia as a terminal disease. In turn, approaches aimed at treatment and cure beyond a point where it is largely in the best interests of the individual have prevailed.

The types of aggressive medical treatment that people with advanced dementia receive as a result are cardiopulmonary resuscitation, frequent admission to hospital, repeat antibiotic therapy and tube feeding. The rationale behind the application of these aggressive treatments may be to extend life and promote relief from symptoms, but what the research shows is that this rationale is misguided and actually may prevent the application of more appropriate care practices. Once again the medicalisation of dementia care has fostered care approaches that are detrimental to the well-being of individuals with dementia.

In a review of the literature concerning end of life care for nursing home residents with advanced dementia, Volicer (2005) summarises the evidence around the application of aggressive medical treatment for this group. Cardiopulmonary resuscitation is three times less likely to be successful in a person with advanced dementia than one with no dementia or with mild dementia and even where the resuscitation is successful most individuals die within 24 hours. Volicer reflects that those with advanced dementia are more likely to be hospitalised than people without dementia or with mild dementia and that hospitalisation is correlated to a decline in functional ability which does not improve on discharge, with patients often developing increased confusion, anorexia, incontinence and propensity to falling. These problems in turn are likely to be treated by aggressive medical interventions. Intercurrent infections are a common consequence of advanced dementia and are treated with antibiotics. This often necessitates diagnostic tests such as blood tests or X-rays, which in themselves have the potential to cause suffering to individuals with severe dementia who are likely to have little understanding of the need for or the process of such tests. Of further concern is that not only do antibiotics raise the risk of uncomfortable side effects (diarrhoea, rash or gastric disturbance for example) but research reflects that use of antibiotics does not prolong life for individuals with severe dementia and is not necessary for the control of symptoms such as raised temperature and pain.

The rationale for the use of tube feeding includes providing a means to eliminate risk of aspiration pneumonia and to improve nutrition; in reality the research demonstrates neither is achieved by the insertion of a feeding tube. The main forms of medical treatment people with advanced dementia are frequently subject to and what the actual outcomes of these interventions are likely to be are summarized below. It is this level of information that it is important for clinicians to include in consultation with the individual and their family when planning for the future. Doing so makes demands on the clinician because the evidence base is growing by the day and new information likely to be pertinent will become available.

Evidence for Practice

Medically Focused End of Life Care

Aimed at treatment and cure

Cardiopulmonary resuscitation (CPR) to extend life

Hospitalisation to investigate and treat symptoms

Antibiotic therapy for frequent intercurrent infections

Tube feeding to overcome risk of aspiration pneumonia, reduce risk of pressure sores developing and to improve nutritional status

Evidenced outcomes for people with advanced dementia

CPR is three times less likely to be successful and where it is successful the individual often dies within 24 hours

Hospitalisation results in functional decline, including increased confusion, anorexia, incontinence and increased incidence of falls

As a result of the deterioration experienced during hospitalisation individuals are likely to be subject to further medical investigation and procedures

Antibiotic therapy is usually preceded by diagnostic tests that are uncomfortable and frightening and the treatment does not prolong life and is not necessary for symptom control

Tube feeding does not prolong life, reduce risk of aspiration pneumonia or pressure sores or improve nutritional status and it is likely to be an uncomfortable procedure to undergo and to live with

The medicalisation of dementia care does a further disservice to those coming to the end of life because the subjective experience of the individual is very poorly understood. We do not know what it is like to die with advanced dementia. A good example is the evidence now available on the treatment of pain for those with dementia; previously pain was unattended on the premise that because it was not expressed it was not felt. There is now growing consensus supported by an extensive evidence base that people with dementia do experience pain, express that experience and have that expression ignored and misinterpreted as symptomatic of dementia. What the evidence reflects is that many, many people have lived with and died with severe dementia and in severe pain. For clinicians caring for individuals with this level of dementia this is indeed a sobering and mortifying fact, but a fact that can clearly be blamed on a previous lack of understanding of the experience of dementia and particularly the experience of severe dementia. What is required now is that those providing care develop methods of extending their knowledge of what it must be like to die with advanced dementia.

Consider, for example, whether the behaviour of a person could be indicating that they are experiencing pain. Abbey *et al.* (2004) developed a scale for assessing pain in individuals with severe dementia and provided six behavioural indicators of pain. These are vocalisation such as crying, whimpering or groaning, facial expression such as frowning, grimacing or looking frightened, change in body language such as rocking, guarding the body or fidgeting, behavioural change such as refusing to eat and increased confusion, physiological change such as temperature or blood pressure being outside normal limits, perspiring or flushing and physical change such as skin tears, arthritis and contractures. The wealth of research evidence now available and still growing on the experience and treatment of pain in individuals with severe dementia is a good example of our ability to extend our knowledge. What is needed now is for that ability to be extended to all areas and for the specialism to concentrate on asking questions about the whole experience of severe dementia and dying with dementia in order that we can better understand and respond to the needs of the people we care for.

Even a cursory look at how care under the medical model impacts on the experience of those dying with dementia illustrates that in terms of improving quality of life, upholding individual wishes and rights (by acting in their best interests) and reinforcing the person within we are not achieving positive outcomes. Rather, I suggest, we are engaged in a futile struggle to prolong life at the expense of the dignity of the person within, the quality of the life remaining and a potentially good death. The emphasis then is on finding and adopting approaches that can better meet the needs of individuals who are coming to the end of their life with dementia and growing and interpreting research to support developing expertise.

A PALLIATIVE APPROACH TO CARE

A growing acknowledgement of the level and nature of the needs of people living with advanced dementia has led to increased support for the adoption of a palliative approach to caring for people with severe dementia. Hanrahan *et al.* (2001) summarise the common medical problems that people with dementia have and make an argument for the role of palliative care for dementia sufferers. These medical problems include swallowing difficulty, pressure sores, aspiration pneumonia, dehydration and malnutrition. Pain and low mood are also likely to be prevalent together with other age related conditions such as osteoporosis and cardiovascular problems.

Palliative care was initially, and to an extent continues to be, provided for individuals in the terminal stages of cancer where life expectancy is not predicted beyond six months. It might not be immediately apparent that the palliative approach represents a step towards best practice in the care of the person with dementia, given that the point of death is singularly difficult to predict, even in the advanced stages of the disease. Some may even question the wisdom of promoting the adoption of a new philosophy of care when the person centred approach we are striving to see incorporated into practice is still far from integral to all areas. We shall see, however, that the principles of palliative care not only offer positive outcomes for the person with dementia and those close to them but also, as Hughes *et al.* (2004) illustrate, affirm and uphold the principles of a person centred approach.

In their briefing on the palliative care needs of older people the National Council for Palliative Care (NCPC) (2006) offers the following definition:

> Palliative care is the active holistic care of patients with advanced progressive illness. Management of pain and other symptoms and provision of psychological, social and spiritual support is paramount. The goal of palliative care is achievement of the best quality of life for patients and their families.

The NCPC, in common with the World Health Organisation (2004b) and many other leading health organisations, now identify that the principles of a palliative care approach should be applied not only to people with cancer but also to people of any age approaching death from any cause in any care setting, in particular older adults and including those who are experiencing dementia. It can readily be seen from the NCPC definition that not only is such an approach applicable to the care of people with dementia, particularly as the disease reaches the later stages, but palliative principles seek to attend to those aspects of the human condition, and particularly human suffering, that we are striving to address through the pursuit of person centred care. The aims of palliative care and how they may be achieved are outlined below.

Evidence for Practice

The Aims of Palliative Care

To provide the best quality of life possible as people approach the end of life

To attend to the individual's emotional, physical, psychological and spiritual needs

To control symptoms of the disease, particularly pain

To provide support and care for those close to the individual

The aims of palliative care may be achieved by

Affirming life and regarding death as a normal process

Not hastening nor postponing death

Providing a support system to enable individuals to live as actively as possible for as long as possible

Offering assistance in achieving specific life goals, for example completing meaningful projects, putting emotional and financial affairs in order

Enabling a life review

Preserving dignity and esteem

Integrating psychological and spiritual care

Providing support and help for family carers to cope during the illness

Control of symptoms including physical, psychological and psychiatric symptoms

Assist at the end of life by attending to suffering (physical, emotional, interpersonal and spiritual)

Responding to needs

Providing support for the family during bereavement

Both palliative care and person centred care seek to place the individual with the disease in a central controlling position with regard to their life. Both adopt an holistic approach in addressing needs and ensuring the best quality of life possible for as long as possible and both recognise the importance of attending to the needs of those close to the individual.

While it may be true that the principles of palliative care are consistent with the employment of a person centred approach, the application of palliative approaches undoubtedly presents a new challenge to clinicians and there are barriers to be overcome. Sachs *et al.* (2004) identify barriers to excellent end of life care for people with dementia that reduce the likelihood of their receiving palliative care, including difficulty in assessing and managing symptoms and difficulty in understanding the caregiver experience and the view that dementia is not a terminal disease. The result is that people with severe dementia often die without adequate pain relief, having been subject to frequent invasive and uncomfortable procedures that have brought little tangible reward. In order to overcome these barriers there is a need for practitioners to understand the issues of living and dying with advanced dementia, developing a specialist ability to assess and treat symptoms (including pain, anxiety, depression, hallucinations, aggression and shouting), developing processes of consulting with individuals and their families, providing practical, emotional and psychological support to enable optimum quality of life and providing bereavement services.

The adoption of a palliative approach to care of people dying with dementia seems to offer a valuable way forward and a significant improvement on the medical model. However, if we consider the aims and objectives as outlined in the previous Evidence for Practice we have to give consideration to the question raised by Shuster (2006), namely: 'Is palliative care best viewed as holistic, person-centred care for persons with chronic illness that begins at the point of diagnosis?' In other words, there is a case for applying palliative care approaches throughout the trajectory of the disease, from the point of diagnosis to the point of death, and, with respect to the family, beyond the point of death.

This may certainly be appropriate if we consider that unlike many other chronic or terminal disease states dementia brings experiences from the point of onset that in other illnesses are associated with the very final stages of the disease, frequently the last three to six months. For example, grief is a condition many people with dementia live with from the point of diagnosis as progressive and relentless loss becomes part of their lives: loss of abilities, loss of independence, loss of friends, esteem and roles. This loss is not confined to the person but affects those close to them – families and friends who must face the point at which their loved one no longer seems to recognise them or be able to correctly name them, the point at which they must accept outside help or take responsibility for the person moving into full-time nursing care or make decisions that affect life quality and quantity. Thus for individuals with dementia and those close to them support with grief is not confined to loss of life but is more likely to be an ongoing process. Similarly, in order to establish the person's preferences for living and dying with advanced dementia we must consult from the point of diagnosis and plan for a time potentially years ahead. It may well be appropriate to take a palliative approach to caring for people with dementia from the onset of the disease.

Caring for people who have dementia is a process that begins at the point of diagnosis and continues to the point of death. The philosophy and approaches that we, as carers, bring to our caring should be fluent and consistent. Thus it makes sense that the aims of palliative care, those of achieving the benefits of disclosing a diagnosis of dementia (discussed in Chapter 4) and the aims of promoting quality of life for persons with dementia (discussed in Chapter 7) share common elements. Incorporating these elements into our practice will enable us to practise in a more person centred way.

The area of research concerned with the experience of severe dementia and dying with dementia is very new. There is certainly great interest in palliation as representing a positive step forward, but more needs to be done in the field of gathering and interpreting evidence. There is also a need to refine our current understanding of palliative care specifically for people with dementia. We should acknowledge that it is unlikely that existing specialist palliative care teams and hospice facilities will expand (both from a capacity and education perspective) to meet the needs of a growing population with dementia. It is more likely that there will be a drive from those currently specialist in caring for people with dementia that will lead to the development of the skills and facility for meeting this need. This in turn is likely to be best facilitated by working with other palliative care specialists to develop pathways of care that fit the needs of individuals with dementia. The elements of a palliative approach to care of people with dementia are given below.

Evidence for Practice

Proposed Elements for a Palliative Approach to Dementia Care

Commences at the point of diagnosis

Incorporates a person centred approach

Involves consultation with the individual with dementia and those close to them

Informs that consultation process with timely and relevant information to enable advance planning and decision making

Offers assistance in achieving specific life goals, for example completing meaningful projects, putting emotional and financial affairs in order

Enables life review

Anticipates and responds to needs

Provides emotional and psychological support, including grief services, throughout the course of the disease

Provides a support system to enable individuals and their carers to live at home for as long as they wish

Provides proactive specialist assessment of symptoms

Provides expert treatment of symptoms based on knowledge of the effects of treatment for individuals with dementia

Provides expert assessment of an individual's levels of well-being, particularly in severe dementia, in order to ensure the individual's desires have the best chance of being considered in the decision making process

Provides bereavement support for family or those close to the individual following death

---

CONCLUSION

In his seminal work on dementia care Professor Kitwood (1997) described the real aim of providing care as being 'to maintain personhood through the entire process of dementia, and to enable a peaceful and person-centred death'. There is no doubt that this aim is under threat from many areas. There is evidence that abuse of people with dementia, particularly at the hands of those charged with their protection and care, is at a worrying level. There is continued evidence that people with dementia are dying in pain and subject to aggressive medical treatments that reap little benefit and have the potential to cause suffering.

There is evidence that a growth in research into the experience of living and dying with advanced dementia is providing tangible means of improving that experience, a good example of this being the development in recognition and management of pain for people with advanced dementia. There is support also for seeking and applying more appropriate methods of care, such as learning from the experts in end of life care, those who provide palliative care for people with cancer. As with virtually every other aspect of caring for people who have dementia we are at that threshold where the evidence is indicating ways forward, more evidence is desperately needed and methods of enabling the translation of that evidence into practice in every area where people with dementia are cared for is urgently required. This is obviously no small task and no doubt Professor Kitwood would be disappointed to see just how long it is taking to generate real change in the speciality. It is, however, the enormity of the challenge and the knowledge that care can be so much better that makes this such an exciting time to be involved in caring for people with dementia.

10 Moving Forward

INTRODUCTION

An explosion of interest in dementia over the past two decades has generated research evidence that demands new approaches to care and, indeed, that requires a metamorphosis in care. The man in the street has a completely new frame of reference for dementia. Although he might call it Alzheimer's disease, people diagnosed with dementia can justifiably expect to have opportunities and to hold expectations for their future that bear no resemblance to the prospects of those living with dementia prior to the 1990s. Drug companies are beginning to unlock the mysteries of the processes of some of the dementias and to offer realistic forms of treatment, with the prospect of cure almost tangible at some point in the near future. Researchers in the fields of medicine, psychology, behaviour, sociology, demography, genetics, technology and nursing are among the many disciplines actively and excitedly investigating and, as we have seen, offering evidence for the way in which policy, services and care can be transformed to benefit those living with dementia and those who will develop it in the future.

We have evidence that challenges many of the presumptions that underpinned traditional approaches to care and research that confirms the right, necessity and ability of people with dementia to be partners in the care process. This should be a time when all involved in the dementia care specialism celebrate success, take satisfaction from their work and actively look for opportunities to further improve care. Dementia care today should look very different when compared with dementia care 20 years ago. This chapter seeks to determine the extent to which changes in the evidence base have infiltrated the world of dementia care and whether improvements in care practice have made the prospect of living with dementia any easier to contemplate. This chapter also considers the particular problem of leading change in 24-hour institutional care.

EVIDENCE OF PROGRESS

Attempts to determine whether or not new research information is infiltrating the world of dementia care and positively influencing the lives of people with dementia is made difficult by a lack of studies in this area. However, two conclusions can hesitantly be drawn from the evidence that is available: firstly, people with early stage dementia are much more likely to be involved in influencing both their own lives and the lives of people with dementia as a whole as a result of the incorporation of new information into care practice and, secondly, the vast majority of people in the later stages of dementia who live in 24-hour care environments continue to experience poor standards of care. For this latter group the evidence base has yet to be translated into positive outcomes.

It would seem that the efforts being made to consult with people who are in the early stages of their dementia are beginning to be effective and the voice of people with dementia is beginning to be heard. This is demonstrated most effectively in the fight for the availability of antidementia drugs. The views of people with dementia are instrumental in the campaign organised by the Alzheimer's Society (2006) to put pressure on the National Institute for Health and Clinical Excellence. Whether these efforts eventually improve the availability of these drugs or not, this working together with people with dementia would have been unthinkable 20 years ago and indicates that a major shift in approach has taken place. The work of Pratt and Wilkinson (2001) is among those leading the way in adding the voice of people with dementia to the debate on diagnosis disclosure. The fact that this voice is contributing to changes in the way diagnosis disclosure is being managed by an increasing number of clinicians demonstrates that a radical change to the way people with early stage dementia are viewed as partners in influencing care has occurred. Indeed, the fact that people with dementia could be included in research would have been considered ridiculous two decades ago; today there are books directing researchers on how to involve people with dementia in their research. People in the early stages of dementia have a growing voice in what happens to them as the professions providing services are beginning to acknowledge what the evidence base is showing: that consultation is possible and service user involvement is critical to the success of service development, operation and evaluation. Professional behaviour is beginning to change in this area to the benefit of people with dementia.

Most people in the early stages of dementia live in their own homes and often have the support of spouse and family. They frequently retain a good ability to communicate and make their wishes and desires known with relative ease. However, a large proportion of people with dementia reside in 24-hour institutional care settings and the evidence for positive change in the life quality of this group is no cause for optimism. Although there are some startling examples of the positive influence of the application of the evidence base these are generally single case, anecdotal examples and there is little evidence of their sustainability. While there may be guidance on how to broaden their application to other care environments there is no evidence that this happens. Such examples are found with regularity on the pages of periodicals like the *Journal of Dementia Care* and to a lesser extent nursing and social care journals. On the positive side this indicates that many practitioners remain keen not only to try and apply evidence to their practice but to share their individual successes to benefit others.

The type of facilities that provide institutional care for people with dementia are residential homes, nursing homes and hospitals, the latter now accounting for less than 5% of places as the last of the large psychiatric hospitals close their doors. There are no definitive numbers for the population with dementia living in 24-hour care settings. Although we may count the number of places specifically available for people with dementia we cannot calculate how many people occupying places for other reasons also have dementia, those who develop dementia once placed into care or indeed those who are never diagnosed. What we can be sure of is that we are talking about hundreds of thousands of people and the numbers are rising. Comas-Herrera *et al.* (2003) cite figures of 227,000 people with cognitive impairment living in institutional care and predict that this figure will rise by 63 % to 365,000 by 2031. Taking into account the difficulty of estimating real numbers we must consider this a conservative estimate.

All of this points to the importance of getting dementia care right and ensuring that what we are learning about the experience of dementia and the needs it generates is incorporated into practice. Ballard *et al.* (2001) provide sobering evidence that not only is institutional care not providing good quality care but that 'radical change' and 'much improvement' is required. In investigating the standards of care for people with dementia in seven National Health Service (NHS) and 10 private care facilities Ballard *et al.* found that involvement in activities, other than being placed in front of a television, absorbed 3% of residents' days, a mere 12 minutes. Residents were communicated with for 50 minutes, representing 14 % of their day, while 30 % of the residents' day was spent in a state of withdrawal where the resident was doing nothing at all. Ballard *et al.* concluded that no facility demonstrated even a 'fair' standard of care and that the results were likely to be representative of the larger picture of institutional care. Indeed, Ward *et al.* (2005) present similar findings with the subjects of their study spending 10 % of their day socially engaged, only 2% of that with care staff.

In the light of what we know about the needs of individuals with dementia we must consider that such figures reflect a neglectful approach to be endemic. Bender and Wainwright (2004) worryingly suggest that the potential for neglect is widespread in institutional care settings and they consider it appropriate to move away from the traditional tendency to blame instances of abuse on one or more evil perpetrators saying it is more likely that systemic weaknesses cause such events. They also suggest that a root-cause analysis would reveal that the devalued status of older people in care is the source of the problem; furthermore, their marginalised position in society means that they are inevitably and permanently at risk of mistreatment.

It could be speculated that change is possible, indeed probable, in the area of early stage dementia care because this process of devaluation occurs once the person is institutionalised. Prior to this they are still viewed as having some value as members of their community or family and may retain the ability to challenge professional behaviour that threatens their personhood. In addition, and crucially perhaps, once professionals begin to apply research to practice the opportunities presented to people in the early stages of dementia and their demonstrable ability to grasp and benefit from these opportunities gives professionals firsthand evidence from their own practice that is powerful enough to quickly embed new approaches and to perpetuate further advances in care.

However, there is little indication that the care people with dementia receive in institutional units is universally benefiting from new information generated by research. Indeed we can only concur with Ward *et al.* (2005) when they conclude that:

> If it is accepted that the key concerns when caring for a person with dementia include support to uphold a sense of self and a social identity and opportunities to maintain a degree of biographical continuity, our study makes clear that institutionalised dementia care is failing service users.

What is reassuring is that some positive change is occurring and this provides hope because we can learn from this. What is also reassuring is that the factors preventing improvement of care in institutional settings are beginning to be understood and thus work to overcome barriers to the absorption of evidence in practice can begin in earnest.

BARRIERS TO INCORPORATING EVIDENCE INTO CARE IN INSTITUTIONAL SETTINGS

The initial belief was that once care staff became aware, in sufficient numbers, of the new evidence and associated theories, in particular the work of Professor Kitwood (1997), together with information on the negative consequences of some of their accustomed practices, they would immediately cease contributing to a negative social psychology and be transformed into better dementia care practitioners. That this has not happened has proved both disappointing and puzzling, for why would one want to persist with practices one has learned are to the detriment of those in one's care? And why would one not want to respond to new needs one has learnt exist?

The answer probably lies in several areas, some of which are related to staff and the way they are managed, some to the way facilities are organised and some to broader issues such as a perceived abdication of its responsibilities by the NHS, loss of meaning through familiarity with the term 'person centred care' and probably the unrealistic expectations that many (including myself) harboured 15 years ago concerning the ease with which the transformation could occur.

As Kitwood (1997) identified, a change of culture is required, which was never going to be achieved overnight. The culture we are attempting to replace, based on a medical approach, has existed as the unchallenged method of care practice for over 100 years. The priorities of care in this model are that the patient is well cared for and safe and the caring practices are primarily and almost exclusively physical and require no input from the recipient of care. Institutional care units are organised to ensure efficiency in achieving these priorities, from the numbers of staff employed to their hours of work and the number and nature of the tasks expected of them during those hours.

In pursuit of a change in care culture, staff are now expected to behave in radically different ways and to accept facts about the capabilities of people with dementia that are not only new to them but are unproven in their own experience. Not only this, but those previously considered among the best practitioners, those who could complete washing, dressing, feeding and toileting tasks most efficiently and those who were able to hold themselves aloof from emotional attachment to those in their care (other than adopting pet names for them) were suddenly informed that not only was this approach to care of people with dementia no longer considered good but actually is now deemed detrimental! We can hardly wonder that the reaction from many such practitioners, rather than to suffer an indignity to their own well-being, is to disregard the evidence and continue as usual. This might not have had such a catastrophic effect if these staff had not been the very people charged with inducting and training the majority of new staff.

Bender and Wainwright (2004) summarise research that reflects the high likelihood of new staff adopting the behaviour of existing staff, even if this is contrary to their own values. Furthermore, they add that obedience is a characteristic of staff in institutional settings; staff do as they are requested or expected to. This suggests that those who hold senior positions are colluding in poor practice and can account for the failure of training, in particular where that training is away from the unit or is academic in nature, because once the newly trained staff return to the unit they revert to expected behaviour within a short period of time. Zimmerman *et al.* (2005), in investigating the attitudes of staff working with people with dementia, found that those working one to two years in 24-hour care settings were more likely to be hopeful and to hold person centred attitudes in their approach than those who had worked longer. They urged that these staff needed support and training to ensure they both stayed in the job and remained positive. Significantly Zimmerman *et al.* also found that staff who perceived themselves to be well trained in dementia care were not only more likely to practice in person centred ways but also to be more satisfied with their work. This has important implications because staff who are satisfied with their work are more likely to be retained, to have lower levels of absenteeism and to be more motivated in providing good quality of care. It can be concluded that the role of the manager and senior staff is vital in determining whether or not a person centred approach will pervade the care area.

While the evidence concerning the nature of the quality of dementia care in institutional settings suggests that overall it is poor and that staff appear to be accountable, we must look beyond this superficial explanation and consider how the organisation of most 24-hour care settings leave the majority of staff with little choice in the way they carry out their care. In fact, many staff make attempts to do more than provide physical care but feel thwarted by the system they must work within. Ward *et al.* (2006) found that staff felt compelled to provide a certain type of care but were aware this was not the type of care they would provide in the ideal world. The quality of care that can be provided is governed by the way care homes are organised and we have repeatedly seen that the priority traditionally lies in ensuring that physical needs are met. Thus staff have to complete the cycle previously described by Ward *et al.* (2005): 'Out of bed–wash–dress–feed–toilet–back to bed' and there is little or no allowance from the perspective of time, resources or support for activity not concerned with fulfilling these basic functions. Despite this, Ward *et al.* concluded that there seems to be an inner dimension to the world of care staff that involves attempting to make sense of the emotional communication of people with dementia but that there is no support for or recognition of this. Staff themselves overlook the importance of this communication and their communication about residents still, Ward *et al.* report, focuses on their physical needs and tasks. Therefore the organisation of care settings does not reflect or facilitate the incorporation of new knowledge, but is this entirely surprising? We have already seen that there is a large section of the population with dementia residing unacknowledged in these services. Can we expect staff, their managers or the owners to identify and translate research to practice to benefit people with dementia in their homes if they are ignorant of the fact that they are there?

MacDonald and Dening (2002) find that, with three-quarters of the population of residential and nursing homes having dementia, dementia care is now their main business. They accuse both the NHS and Social Services of avoiding dementia and suggest that such avoidance has implications for staffing levels, training and support of staff in most homes; as these are key components of quality care there is great cause for concern. They state that the need to improve dementia awareness and care skills among not only care staff but inspection and registration staff, hospitals, purchasers and politicians is now urgent. Bender and Wainwright (2004) also point out that with increasing numbers being cared for in the private sector the progressively higher standards demanded by the inspectorate will mean that in order for home owners to maximise their profit corners will inevitably be cut, meaning lower staff to resident ratios, poorer pay for staff and poor maintenance of buildings or environments, none of which is conducive to dynamic and progressive care.

Neither is the organisation of care through provision of specialist dementia care units problem free. Such units are primarily occupied by people with severe dementia with challenging behaviour, meaning that those with such behaviour may benefit from specialist intervention but those with severe dementia who sit quietly in other settings where staff perceive them as placid and easy to care for have no access to specialist care. Some commentators have also highlighted that the stress levels of staff working in specialised units is high, indicating that working with people with severe dementia is very stressful. We need to consider in whose interest it is to assemble people with severe dementia into group living and whether there are better ways to organise care or support staff in these situations.

One aspect of the new dementia care culture that certainly seems to have permeated practice settings is the language of care. Organisations from the Department of Health, with their *National Service Framework for Older People* (2001a), to individual nursing homes in their promotional leaflets recognise the advantage of using the new terminology. However, the accusation is that rather than being indicative of an overall change in care culture this is merely proof that we have learned to 'talk the talk'. In fact, the ability of social, health and private care services to use the language may be masking the real extent of the lack of change thus far achieved. The term 'person centred care' has become so overused that in respect of what it means to care for an individual with dementia, as Professor Kitwood intended, it has become diluted to the point of being meaningless.

Many now working in dementia care can say that person centred care involves treating people as individuals and encouraging choice. Of course it does, but the philosophy and application with regard to people who have dementia and in illustrating what needs to change for care to be good this term is something infinitely richer and more demanding. When Sheard (2004) likens person centred care to the story of the Emperor's new suit, in that everyone has heard of it but no one has seen it, it is hard to disagree.

Evidence for Practice

Barriers to Incorporating Evidence into Care in Institutional Settings

The priorities of traditional care are firmly embedded into practice by rigid organisational systems

The evidence highlights the inadequacies of traditional care and carers by association; this, together with a lack of firsthand experience of the positive outcomes possible, has led to carers denying the evidence

Peer pressure leads to new staff adopting existing practice or leaving

New staff need support and further training to continue to hold positive person centred views; this is not forthcoming

Nearly 75 % of the residents in care homes have dementia; this is not acknowledged by governing bodies within health and social care and perpetuates poor allocation of resources

Overuse of the term 'person centred care' has devalued the real meaning of it in terms of the needs of people with dementia

The vast majority of care is now provided by the private sector where the demand for high standards of care increasingly eats into profit margins and in turn encourages home owners to cut corners to maximise profit

---

OVERCOMING BARRIERS TO INCORPORATING EVIDENCE INTO CARE IN INSTITUTIONAL SETTINGS

When we talk about incorporating the evidence base into care practice it is quite clear that the level of change required is a change in the culture of care. Thus we are primarily talking about changing the values held by carers and the behaviour these values espouse, expressed as care practices and the structures that facilitate them. We want the values to change from those expressed in the attitudes described above that see people with dementia as valueless and support care practices that prioritise physical care and efficiency. We want to instil values that reflect care staff acceptance of people with dementia as valuable human beings who contribute to the community and retain the ability to improve the quality of their lives. There is hope that this is possible. There are examples of staff groups who are motivated and achieve positive outcomes. Staff new to dementia care seem to arrive with a positive attitude and good levels of motivation. Other research shows that job satisfaction is higher among those who perceive they provide good quality care (Zimmerman *et al.* 2005; Castle *et al.* 2006) and, as Ward *et al.* (2005) report, some staff want and indeed attempt to provide more than basic care. Finally, if peer pressure encourages staff to conform to traditional practices then it is highly likely that if practice changes to a more positive approach then this peer pressure will help sustain improvement. However, none of these potentially positive changes will occur spontaneously; change needs to be driven.

The key element of this drive for change will be neither money nor an increase in staff. Although both would be invaluable it is not realistic to expect either at this point in time. This should not deter us from continuing to be vociferous in demanding more resources but neither should it take our focus from what can be achieved within the resources we currently have. There is one element necessary in the drive for change, arguably the most important element, which is readily available in each care facility in the country – a potential change agent, the facility manager.

Most managers come up through the ranks and have little or no management training (Johnson *et al.* 1999). This presents not only the obvious problems with regard to the level of management competency but also raises concern that internal promotion may mean the manager is quite likely to be immersed in the existing culture. This may make it both difficult to recognise the need for change and difficult to implement change should they wish to. However, individuals in management positions in care homes do not fall into them by accident and the vast majority want to instigate and support positive change, they want to do a good job. Unless the importance of the role of managers is recognised, supported and celebrated the status quo will continue. Those recruiting to positions of management of our homes need to understand the importance of skills in change management and leadership.

Managers in 24-hour care settings need to take responsibility for leading the team of staff and for introducing, incorporating and sustaining the influence of the evidence base in the facilities that they manage. The management role is the key to the implementation and maintenance of any change in the way a unit operates. Whatever resources are available, the manager can make the difference between good and poor care. A poor manager can squander and misalign financial and other resources whereas a good manager will work with what there is in order to achieve positive results and where this is difficult will seek further resources appropriately.

The most important resource that any manager has at their disposal is the staff team. Investing in the team, building the team and responding to individuals within the team in a person centred way will build an expectation that they respond to those in their care in a person centred way.

Cantley and Wilson (2002) identify effective management strategies that have been shown to produce high quality care homes for people with dementia, including ensuring that all staff have specific knowledge, skills and commitment for dementia care, staffing levels that allow for individual attention for residents, providing appropriate support for staff undertaking this emotionally demanding work, involving relatives and residents with dementia not only in influencing individual care but in the way the home is run and maintaining good links with local resources. The World Health Organization (http://www.who.int/employment/competencies/en/) summarises some of the more common competencies associated with good management, including good communication, fostering teamwork, setting an example and empowering staff. Bearing these competencies and strategies in mind, the manager is charged with both managing and leading the team to develop and deliver good quality care.

Norris-Baker *et al.* (2003) describe an effective process of managing culture change in homes that commences with simply asking the staff group: 'What would this home have to be like for you to be happy living here?' Asking staff to define and document what the ideal nursing home would be like is also a start. Team discussions can facilitate the definition of a philosophy and set of beliefs about care that the team are happy to subscribe to, these become the underpinning ideals that dictate team practice and activity. It is during these discussions that the manager introduces the evidence base, information about the experience of dementia and the needs people with dementia are likely to have, and indeed explores ways in which staff can uncover more about each individual's needs.

The biggest obstacle to initiating change may prove to be the killer statements some long term members of the team employ, such as 'we tried that before and it doesn't work'. The manager needs to be strong to overcome not only such statements but the undermining effect such statements can bring if individual staff members translate their objections into obstructive practices, for example refusing to do certain things, encouraging other staff to refuse or behaving differently when the manager is not in attendance. This highlights the need for the manager to be a visible presence, but also presents the manager with an opportunity. If the manager can predict those who are likely to try and obstruct change then they can be singled out for special responsibility. Prior to introducing the subject of change the manager can draw this member of the team aside and pre-empt their objection, perhaps by saying 'I know we've tried this before, but . . . ' and going on to explain why it can succeed now and asking for specific help from the staff member. It may be through such approaches that the manager can turn a potential obstruction into a positive aid. Another obstacle the manager must overcome is that of time, the traditional espoused enemy of providing activities and increased communication for residents. Indeed, the manner in which care is organised traditionally means that once personal care, toilet requirements and dietary needs are seen to and records updated there appears little time for anything other than a brief break for staff away from the client group to recoup energy. To identify just what is being done with time a detailed picture of a day in the life of the home can be compiled. This involves charting how staff spend their time from the beginning of a shift to the end, recording how many minutes it takes for tasks to be accomplished with each client and how many staff contribute, and how long other non-resident-contact tasks take. For example, if it takes two staff 15 minutes to help Mrs Bloggs to wash and dress this is recorded as 30 minutes per day, if it takes one member of staff 40 minutes to feed Mr Jones and he eats three times a day the activity accounts for 2 hours per day, or if it takes two staff 10 minutes to take Mrs Smith to the toilet and this is done five times a day the task accounts for 100 minutes. Charting the care hours in this way it becomes easy to see both where the time goes and how much time, if any, is spare. Obviously if spare time is found it can be used to provide for the psychosocial needs of the individuals cared for. If no spare time is found the manager should lead the team in considering the importance of the activities that are not care based, such as record keeping, sorting laundry, cleaning and tidying, and whether these tasks could be done differently to maximise time for attending to psychosocial needs of those in their care. A further discussion of each client from the perspective of how their needs are currently met and how their care could be rearranged to allow for social and relationship opportunities is necessary. For example, does Mrs Smith need to go to the toilet five times a day? If she were taken only four times a surplus of 20 minutes per day is available to do something else. In a study of the well-being among people with dementia in long term care Bruce *et al.* (2002) found that, if residents were aware that something interesting would happen sooner or later, they were able to tolerate a degree of boredom. Furthermore, they observed that once stimulation was provided residents had the capacity to come to life. In this context finding an extra 20 minutes per day to spend in stimulating activity with Mrs Smith is vital. Once the philosophy and beliefs of the team are described part of instilling the new practices would be about how different care tasks are prioritised for individual clients. Finding minutes for each resident will become paramount and staff will then need support and encouragement to develop and use skills in meeting psychosocial needs, to learn to communicate in meaningful ways that support identity and to undertake life story work, reminiscence, games or musical activities that will begin to address the psychological needs of those in their care.

The manager certainly needs to be able to interpret the evidence base. Managers need to know their facts in order to recognise the direction they should be going and to support their teams in the development. Frequently this is interpreted as a need for training and frequently this training is expensive. This is problematic because funding for training is restricted across both the private and public sectors. Even when funds are available there may be confusion on how best to spend it. However, given the depth and breadth of information that is available for minimum investment or even free of charge through the Internet, subscription to the right journals, access to a decent library or through voluntary organisations such as the Alzheimer's Society, this need not be a big problem. What funds are available are possibly best spent initially on giving managers the skills to interpret the evidence base and to manage and lead their teams. The manager can then take responsibility for training team members, demonstrating good practice on a daily basis themselves and celebrating success with the team, thus embedding what is being learned into the culture of the home's care.

Misiorski (2003) describes four critical elements to achieving change in the nursing home culture: firstly, the getting ready stage, involving clarifying the purpose and values of the home; secondly, the implementation stage, during which practices and the behaviour of staff are aligned with the purpose and values; thirdly, evaluation wherein the action and outcomes thereof are reviewed; lastly, defining where to go next, which involves celebrating success and moving on. At each stage the skill and leadership of the manager will be critical.

What is needed, as Haseman (2004) identifies, is a style of leadership that encourages high quality care rather than one that simply deters poor quality. This style of management is authoritarian, not in the stereotypical sense of being overbearing or dictatorial but in a manner that consults with team members and analyses what they say along with information from the evidence base to come to the correct decision about a course of action. Through delegating and directing the leader begins to shape practice and through recognition and celebration of success the leader reinforces and progresses the quality of care. The style of leadership may change as the team develops and matures but a large amount of delegation and instruction is likely to prompt success initially. What is required of those managing and leading change in institutional care settings is highlighted at the end of the section.

Changing the way we behave towards people with dementia in our care homes can be as difficult or as easy as we make it. Plenty of money and additional resources will help and will be necessary in the future, but will not resolve the underlying cause of poor quality care if we agree with Bender and Wainwright (2004) that the cause is the devalued status we attach to those in our care. Institutional dementia care now needs to move from the medical arena where physical care is the pinnacle to the specialist arena, where the meeting of physical care needs is a given and the emphasis is on sustaining an individual's identity, celebrating their life and ensuring their empowerment and agency within the context of their lives and future. We urgently need leaders with the ability and motivation to lead the required change but we also need to recognise errors in policy and systemic weakness that foster the type of environments that make change difficult.

Evidence for Practice

Managing and Leading Change in Institutional Care Settings

The role of leading, sustaining and managing change is a function of the person charged with managing a care facility

A good leader recognises that the most important resource they have at their disposal is the staff team

A good manager understands that investing in the team, building the team and responding to individual members of the team in a person centred way is the basis for expecting staff to respond to people with dementia in a similar way

A good manager will take responsibility for introducing evidence to practice and enabling the team to incorporate it into daily practice

A good leader will anticipate and act to overcome the obstacles individual team members may present; doing this in a positive manner can contribute to success

A good manager will lead by example as a visible and positive role model

A good leader will celebrate success and realise that it can breed success

A good leader will consult with staff and balance their views with information from the evidence base prior to acting

CONCLUSION

The demands required to put research into practice have significantly outstripped the ability of many organisations providing care for people with dementia to translate this research into practice. This has led experts in the area to question the extent to which as a specialism we have achieved anything approaching the new culture of care that Kitwood (1997) claimed was required. The specialism stands accused of developing nothing more than a new language.

The dementia care specialism is huge. People with dementia live in many places, cross several generation spans, exist in various and contrasting cultural and social circumstances with multiple and complex group and individual needs. Those who provide services for them range from familial and informal carers across a wide and diverse range of professional and voluntary organisations and disciplines. At the national level the Government, National Health Service, Social Services and the Alzheimer's Society are involved in trying to direct the path of care, driven in turn by an enormous surge in the research and developmental base which increasingly reveals that what has previously passed for 'care' is at best misdirected and at worst abusive. Professional carers, in the space of 20 years, have been expected to transform from those from whom only basic physical care skills were required to the highly skilled practitioners needed to meet the needs of people with dementia that the research has uncovered. Given that the research largely presents outcomes rather than solutions, that the spectrum across which the change must occur is huge and that a lowly status has been afforded the elderly in our society together with a lack of resource allocation, the wonder is not that the transformation is not complete but that we have come as far as we have.

If a measure of a society is the manner in which it treats its most vulnerable members the way in which people with dementia are treated within our society reflects poorly upon us. Ageist attitudes continue to deny people with dementia the places, staff, training, funding, protection and basic human respect that are required to deliver the changes that research confirms are desperately and urgently needed. The harsh but true reality is that with increased life expectancy many of us will develop dementia.

When we do or those close to us do we will begin to appreciate the value of investment in services for people with dementia. By that point it will be too late.

In many respects it feels as though dementia care is at a crossroad; it can become a dynamic specialism responsive to new evidence and new ideas where the prospect of a diagnosis of dementia, while life altering, can be managed with hope or it can stagnate or, worse, deteriorate further as the growth in the older population generates ever-increasing demands on a service unable to cope through a lack of resources, understanding or desire. If society has a role in determining the progress of the dementia care specialism then as an individual we each have a role: firstly, as members of society who contribute to and help shape the society we live in by pressuring those in positions of influence nationally, locally and within the services that are available and, secondly, through the relationships we foster with people who have dementia.

The very least we can do is meet and communicate with people who have dementia as individuals with compassion and kindness, with interest and empathy. In our busy working life, particularly in 24-hour care settings, we can find some extra minutes to communicate about something other than our need to complete a physical task with the person. We can at least take the time to discover personally whether the research is right and people with dementia, even severe dementia, continue to want and to seek contact with us. If you have not already discovered this be prepared to be surprised and then shamed by the times you have not acknowledged this. Hopefully the team you work within will support you in resolving to do things differently or maybe you will be the agent of change who focuses your team on the need to do things differently.

References

Abbey, J., Piller, N., De Bellis, A., Esterman, A., Parker, D., Giles, L., & Lowcay, B. (2004) The Abbey pain scale: a 1-minute numerical indicator for people with end-stage dementia. *International Journal of Palliative Nursing,* **10**(1), 6–13.

Adams, K., & Sanders, S. (2004) Alzheimer's caregiver differences in experience of loss, grief reactions and depressive symptoms across stage of disease. *Dementia,* **3**(2), 195–210.

Alexopoulos, G., Abrams, R., Young, R., & Shanoian, C. (1988) Cornell scale for depression in dementia. *Biological Psychiatry,* **23**, 271–84.

Allan, K. (2001) *Communication and Consultation: Exploring Ways for Staff to Involve People with Dementia in Developing Services,* The Policy Press, Bristol.

Almberg, B., Grafstrom, M., & Wimblad, B. (1997) Major strain and coping strategies as reported by family members who care for aged demented relatives. *Journal of Advanced Nursing,* **26**(4), 683–91.

Altschul, A., & Simpson, R. (1957) *Psychiatric Nursing,* Bailliere Tindall, London.

Altschul, A., & Simpson, R. (1977) *Psychiatric Nursing,* 5th edn, Bailliere Tindall, London.

Alzheimer's Society (2004) *Celebrating the Last 25 Years,* Annual Review 2003/2004, Gordon House, London.

Alzheimer's Society (2006) [online], available: http://www.alzheimers.org.uk/news_and_campaigns/policy_watch/demography. htm [30 October 2006].

Alzheimer's Society Report (2006) Alzheimer's Society response to NICE Appraisal consultation document 2 [online], available: http://www.alzheimers.org.uk/news_and_campaigns/PDF/AlzheimersSocietyResponse_NiceACD2_Feb06.pdf [20 August 2006].

Amar, K., & Wilcock, G. (1996) Fortnightly review: vascular dementia. *British Medical Journal,* **312**, 227–31.

Anderson, C., Wittrup-Jensen, K., Lolk, A., Anderson, K., & Kragh-Sorensen, P. (2004) Ability to perform activities of daily living is the main factor affecting quality of life in patients with dementia. *Health and Quality of Life Outcomes* [online], available: http://www.hqlo.com/content/2/1/52 [6 August 2006].

Ballard, C., & Waite, J. (2006) The effectiveness of atypical antipsychotics for the treatment of aggression and psychosis in Alzheimer's disease. *The Cochrane Database of Systematic Reviews,* Issue 1, Art. No.: CD003476. DOI: 10.1002/14651858.CD00 3476.pub2.

Ballard, C., Fossey, J., Chithramohan, R., Howard, R., Burns, A., Thompson, P., Tadros, G., & Fairbairn, A. (2001) Quality of care in private sector and NHS facilities for people with dementia: cross sectional survey. *British Medical Journal,* **323**, 426–7.

Ballard, C., Margallo-Lana, M., Juszczak, E., Douglas, S., Swann, A., Thomas, A., O'Brien, J., Everratt, A., Sadler, S., Maddison, C., Lee, L., Bannister, C., Elvish, R., & Jacoby, R. (2005) Quetiapine and rivastigmine and cognitive decline in Alzheimer's disease: randomised double blind placebo controlled trial. *British Medical Journal,* **330**, 874–77.

Bamford, C., Lamont, S., Eccles, M., Robinson, L., May, C., & Bond, J. (2004) Disclosing a diagnosis of dementia: a systematic review. *International Journal of Geriatric Psychiatry*, **19**, 151–69.

Banerjee, S., Smith, S., Lamping, D., Harwood, R., Foley, B., Smith, P., Murray, J., Prince, M., Levin, E., Mann, A., & Knapp, M. (2006) Quality of life in dementia: more than just cognition. An analysis of associations with quality of life in dementia. *Journal of Neurological and Neurosurgical Psychiatry*, **77**, 146–8.

Barnett, M. (2004) A GP guide to breaking bad news. *Practitioner,* **248**, 392–405.

Bender, M. (2004) *Therapeutic Groupwork for People with Cognitive Losses: Working with People with Dementia*, Speechmark Publishing Limited, Oxford.

Bender, M., & Wainwright, T. (2004) So sad to see good care go bad – but is it surprising? *Journal of Dementia Care,* **12**(5), 27–9.

Biernacki, C., & Barratt, J. (2001) Improving the nutritional status of people with dementia. *British Journal of Nursing*, **10**(17), 1104–14.

Bird, M., Llewellyn-Jones, R., Smithers, H., Andrews, C., Cameron, I., Cottee, A., Hutson, C., Jenneke, B., Kurrle, S., & Russell, B. (1998) Challenging behaviours in dementia: a project at Hornsby/Ku-ring-gai Hospital. *Australian Journal on Ageing*, **17**, 10–15.

Bird, M., Llewellyn-Jones, R., Smither, H., & Korten, A. (2002) Psychosocial approaches to challenging behaviour in dementia: a controlled trial. Report to the Commonwealth of Health and Ageing: Office for Older Australians, Canberra.

Birks, J. (2006) Cholinesterase inhibitors for Alzheimer's disease. *The Cochrane Database of Systematic Reviews*, Issue 1, Art. No.: CD005593. DOI: 10.1002/14651858.CD005593.

Birks, J., & Grimley Evans, J. (2002) Ginkgo biloba for cognitive impairment and dementia. *The Cochrane Database of Systematic Reviews*, Issue 4, Art. No.: CD003120. DOI: 10.1002/14651858.CD003120.

Birks, J., & Harvey, R. (2003) Donepezil for dementia due to Alzheimer's disease. *The Cochrane Database of Systematic Reviews*, Issue 3, Art. No.: CD001190. DOI: 10.1002/14651858.CD001190.

Birks, J., Grimley Evans, J., Iakovidou, V., & Tsolaki, M. (2000) Rivastigmine for Alzheimer's disease. *The Cochrane Database of Systematic Reviews*, Issue 4, Art. No.: CD001191. DOI: 10.1002/14651858.CD001191.

Bourgeois, M. (2003) Using the written word to overcome memory deficits. *Aging, Health and Society: News and View,* **9**(1), 3–4.

Bowling, A., Gabriel, Z., Marriott Dowding, L., Evans, O., Fleissig, A., Banister, D., & Sutton, S. (2003) Let's ask them: a national survey of definitions of quality of life and its enhancement among people aged 65 and over. *International Journal of Aging and Human Development*, **56**(4), 269–306.

Bradford Dementia Group (2005) *DCM 8 User's manual*. University of Bradford, Bradford.

Braudy Harris, P. (2002) The subjective experience of early on-set dementia: voices of the persons. Paper presented to the 55th Gerontological Society of America Annual Meeting.

Briggs Report (1972) *Report on the Committee on Nursing*, HMSO, London.

British Geriatrics Society Compendium. 4.10 Abuse of Older People (April 2005) [online], available: http://www.bgs.org.uk/Publications/Compendium/compend_4–10.htm [accessed 30 May 2006].

Brod, M., Stewert, A., Sands, L., & Walton, P. (1999) Conceptualization and measurement of quality of life in dementia: the dementia quality of life instrument (DQoL). *The Gerontologist*, **39**(1), 25–35.

Brooker, D. (2001) Therapeutic activity, in *A Handbook of Dementia Care* (ed. C. Cantley), Open University Press, Buckingham.

Brooker, D. (2002) Dementia care mapping: a look at its past, present and future. *Journal of Dementia Care*, **10**(3), 33–6.

Brooker, D. (2005) Dementia care mapping: a review of the literature. *The Gerontologist*, **45**, 11–18.

Bruce, E., Surr, C., Tibbs, M., & Downs, M. (2002) Moving towards a special kind of care for people with dementia living in care homes. *NT Research,* **7**(5), 335–47.

Bullock, R. (2005) Treatment of behavioural and psychiatric symptoms in dementia: implications of recent safety warnings. *Current Medical Research and Opinion*, **21**(1), 1–10.

Byrne, P. (2000) Stigma of mental illness and ways of diminishing it. *Advances in Psychiatric Treatment*, **6**, 65–72.

Cantley, C., & Wilson, R. (2002) Designing and managing care homes for people with dementia [online], available: http://www.jrf.org.uk/knowledge/findings/socialcare/312.asp#top [15 September 2006].

Carey, N. (2004) *Celebrating the Last 25 Years. Alzheimer's Society Annual Review 2003/2004,* Gordon House, London.

Carpenter, B., & Dave, J. (2004) Disclosing a dementia diagnosis: a review of opinion and practice, and a proposed research agenda. *The Gerontologist*, **44**, 149–58.

Casarett, D., & Karlawish, J. (1999) Working in the dark: the state of palliative care for patients with severe dementia. *Generations*, **23**(1), 18–23.

Castle, N., Degenholtz, H., & Rosen, J. (2006) Determinants of staff job satisfaction of caregivers at two nursing homes in Pennsylvania. *BMC Health Services Research* [online], available: http://www.biomedcentral.com/1472–6963/6/60 [accessed 27 August 2006].

Cheston, R. (1996) Stories and metaphors: talking about the past in a psychotherapy group for people with dementia. *Ageing and Society*, **16**, 579–602.

Cheston, R., Jones, K., & Gilliard, J. (2003) Group psychotherapy for people with dementia. *Nursing and Residential Care*, **5**(4), 186–8.

Clarfield, A.M. (2003) The decreasing prevalence of reversible dementias: an updated meta-analysis. *Archives of Internal Medicine*, **163**, 2219–29.

Coleman, D. (2001) Population ageing: an unavoidable future. *Social Biology and Human Affairs*, **66**, 1–11.

Comas-Herrera, A., Wittenberg, R., Pickard, L., Knapp, M., & MRCCFAS (2003) Cognitive impairment in older people: its implications for future demand for services and costs. Report to the Alzheimer's Research Trust, PSSRU Discussion Paper (1728).

Commission for Health Improvement (2003) *Investigation into Matters Arising from care on Rowan Ward*, Manchester Mental Health and Social Care Trust, The Stationery Office, London.

Commission for Social Care Inspection (2006) *Handled with Care? Managing Medication for Residents of Care Homes and Children's Homes – A Follow up Study*. The Stationery Office, London.

Committee on Safety of Medicines (2004) Atypical antipsychotic drugs and stroke. Message from Professor Gordon Duff, Chairman, Committee on Safety of Medicines [online], available: http://www.info.doh.gov.uk/doh/embroadcast.nsf/0/ 3d8dbb48b26ff90280256e520045977a?OpenDocument [accessed 20 June 2006].

Cooper, S., & Prasher, V. (1998) Maladaptive behaviours and symptoms of dementia in adults with Down's syndrome compared with adults with intellectual disability of other aetiologies. *Journal of Intellectual Disability*, **42**(4), 293–300.

Cotrell, V., & Schulz, R. (1993) The perspective of the patient with Alzheimer's disease: a neglected dimension of dementia research. *The Gerontologist*, **33**(2), 205–211.

Crisp, A., Gelder, M., Rix, S., Meltzer, H., & Rowlands, O. (2000) Stigmatisation of people with mental illness. *British Journal of Psychiatry*, **177**, 4–7.

Davis, R. (1989) *My Journey into Alzheimer's Disease: A Story of Hope*, Tyndale House, Wheaton, Illinois.

Day, C. (1997) Validation therapy: a review of the literature. *Journal of Gerontological Nursing*, **23**(4), 29–34.

Debate of the Age Health and Care Study Group (1999) *The Future of Health and Care of Older People: The Best Is Yet to Come*, Age Concern, London.

Dent, V. (2003) *Group Activities with Older Adults*, Speechmark Publishing Limited, Oxford.

Department of Health (1990) *The NHS and Community Care Act*, The Stationery Office, London.

Department of Health (1997) *The New NHS: Modern and Dependable*, The Stationery Office, London.

Department of Health (1998) *A First Class Service: Quality in the New NHS*, The Stationery Office, London.

Department of Health (2001a) *National Service Framework for Older People*, The Stationery Office, London.

Department of Health (2001b) *Medicines and Older People: Implementing Medicine-Related Aspects of the NSF for Older People*, The Stationery Office, London.

Department of Health (2002) *Shifting the Balance of Power: The Next Steps,* The Stationery Office, London.

Department of Health (2004) *Guidance for the Protection of Vulnerable Adults (POVA) Scheme* [online], available: www.doh.gov.uk [accessed 31 May 2006].

Department of Health and Home Office (2000) *No Secrets: Guidance on Developing and Implementing Multi-agency Policies and Procedures to Protect Vulnerable Adults from Abuse* [online], available: www.doh.gov.uk [accessed 31 May 2006].

Double, D. (2001) Can psychiatry be retrieved from a biological approach? *Journal of Critical Psychology, Counselling and Psychotherapy*, **1**, 28–31.

Draper, B. (1999) Practical geriatrics: the diagnosis and treatment of depression in dementia. *Psychiatric Services*, **50**, 1151–3.

Erde, E., Nadal, E., & School, T. (1988) On truth telling and the diagnosis of Alzheimer's disease. *Journal of Family Practice*, **26**, 401–6.

Feil, N. (1982) *Validation. The Feil Method. How to Help the Disorientated Old-Old*, Feil Productions, Cleveland.

Feil, N.(1993) *The Validation Breakthrough*, Health Professionals Press, Baltimore.

Fitzpatrick, A., Kuller,L., Lopez, O., Kawas, C., & Jagust, W. (2005) Survival following dementia onset: Alzheimer's disease and vascular dementia. *Journal of the Neurological Sciences,* **229/230**, 43–9.

Foley, K., Sudha, S., Sloane, P., & Gold, D. (2003) Staff perceptions of successful management of severe behavioural problems in dementia special care units. *Dementia*, **2**(1), 105–24.

Folstein, M., Folstein, S., & McHugh, P. (1975) Mini-mental state: a practical method for grading the cognitive state of patients for the clinician. *Journal of Psychiatric Research*, **12**, 189–98.

Forbes, S., Bern-Klug, M., & Gessert, C. (2000) End-of-life decision making for nursing home residents with dementia. *Journal of Nursing Scholarship*, **32**, 251–8.

Freud, S. (1905) *On Psychotherapy*. Reprinted 1953–1974, in *the Standard Edition of the Complete Works of Sigmund Freud* (trans. and ed. J. Strachey), Vol. 7, Hogarth Press, London.

Fromage, B., & Anglade, P. (2002) The ageing of Downs Syndrome subjects. *Encephale*, **28**(3), 212–6.

Galloway, S. (2006) *Quality of Life and Well-being: Measuring the Benefits of Culture and Sport: Literature Review*, Scottish Executive Education Department [online], available: http://www.scotland.gov.uk/Resource/Doc/89281/002(1350)pdf [accessed 17 August 2006].

Garner, J. (2004) Dementia, in *Talking over the Years: A Handbook of Dynamic Psychotherapy with Older People* (eds. S. Evans & J. Garner), Brunner-Routledge, Hove.

Gates, G., Karzon, R., Garcia, P., Peterein, J., Storandt, M., Morris, J., & Miller, J. (1995) Auditory dysfunction in aging and senile dementia of the Alzheimer's type. *Archives of Neurology*, **52**(6), 626–34.

Goldsmith, M. (1996) *Hearing the Voice of People with Dementia: Opportunities and Obstacles*, Jessica Kingsley, London.

Gräsel, E., Wiltfang, J., & Kornhuber, J. (2003) Non-drug therapies for dementia: an overview of the current situation with regard to proof effectiveness. *Dementia and Geriatric Cognitive Disorders*, **14**(3), 115–26.

Hanrahan, P., Luchins, D., & Murphy, K. (2001) Palliative care for patients with dementia, in *Palliative Care for Non-cancer Patients* (eds. J., Addington-Hall & I. Higginson). Oxford University Press, London.

Harper, L., Lyle, A., Moorthy, T., Reddon, J., Brahim, A., & Ward, J. (2004) Depression and challenging behaviors in psychogeriatric patients who have a dementia. *The Gerontologist*, **44**(1), 653.

Haseman, C. (2004) Can administrators leadership style influence quality of care? [online], available: http://www.nursinghomesmagazine.com/Past_Issues.htm?ID=3342 [accessed 2 September 2006].

Health Survey for England (1998) *Cardiovascular Disease*, Vol. 1, *Findings*, The Stationery Office, London.

Hebert, P., Hoffmaster, B., Glass, K., & Singer, P. (1997) Bioethics for clinicians:7. Truth telling. *Canadian Medical Association Journal*, **156** (2), 225–8.

Heller, T., & Heller, L. (2003) First among equals? Does drug treatment for dementia claim more than its fair share of resources? *Dementia*, **2**(1), 7–19.

Hepple, J. (2004) Psychotherapies with older people: an overview. *Advances in Psychiatric Treatment*, **10**, 371–7.

Heston, C. (2002) [online], available: http://transcripts.cnn.com/TRANSCRIPTS/0208/09/bn.09.html [accessed 5 June 2006].

Holland, A., Hon, J., Huppert, F., Stevens, F., & Watson, P. (1998) Population-based study of the prevalence and presentation of dementia in adults with Down's syndrome. *British Journal of Psychiatry*, **172**, 493–8.

Holroyd, S., Snustad, D., & Chalifoux, R. (1996) Attitudes of older adults on being told the diagnosis of Alzheimer's disease. *Journal of the American Geriatrics Society*, **44**, 400–3.

Hopper, T., Bayles, K., Harris, F., & Holland, A. (2001) The relationship between minimum data set ratings and scores on measures of communication and hearing among nursing home residents with dementia. *American Journal of Speech–Language Pathology*, **10**(4), 370–82.

Hudson, S., & Boyter, A. (1997) Pharmaceutical care of the elderly. *The Pharmaceutical Journal,* **259**, 686–8.

Hughes, J., Hedley, K., & Harris, D. (2004) The practice and philosophy of palliative care in dementia. *Nursing and Residential Care*, **6**(1), 27–30.

Hunter, R., & Macalpine, I. (1963) *Three Hundred Years of Psychiatry 1535–1860. A History Presented in Selected English Texts,* Oxford University Press, London.

Jackson, S., Mangoni, A., & Batty, G. (2003) Optimization of drug prescribing. *British Journal of Clinical Pharmacology*, **57**(3), 231–6.

Jacques, A. (1988) *Understanding Dementia*, Churchill Livingstone, London.

Jacques, A.(1992) *Understanding Dementia*, 2nd edn, Churchill Livingstone, Edinburgh.

Johnson, H., Bouman, W., & Pinner, G. (2000) On telling the truth in Alzheimer's disease: a pilot study of current practice and attitudes. *International Psychogeriatrics*, **12**, 221–9.

Johnson, M., Cullen, L., & Patsios, D. (1999) *The Training Needs of Managers of Long-Term Care*, Summary of Findings [online], available: http://www.jrf.org.uk/knowledge/findings/socialcare/pdf/FO19.pdf [accessed 24 August 2006].

Jones, K., Cheston, R., & Gillard, J. (2002) *Group Psychotherapy for People with Dementia. A Dementia Voice Project* [online], available: http://www.dementia-voice.org.uk/Projects/psychotherapyreport.pdf [accessed 5 May 2006].

Katz, S., Down, T., Cash, H., & Grotz, R. (1970) Progress in the development of the index of ADL. *Gerontologist*, **10**, 20–30.

Keady, J. (1996) The experience of dementia: a review of the literature and implications for nursing practice. *Journal of Clinical Nursing*, **5**(5), 275–88.

Keady, J., & Nolan, M. (1994) Younger onset dementia: developing a longitudinal model as the basis for a research agenda and as a guide to interventions with sufferers and carers. *Journal of Advanced Nursing*, **19**(4), 659–69.

Keith, I. (2002) Dementia with Lewy bodies. *British Journal of Psychiatry*, **180**, 144–7.

Killick, J. (2005) Making sense of dementia through metaphor. *Journal of Dementia Care*, **13**(1), 22–3.

Kitwood, T. (1995) Cultures of care: tradition and change, in *The New Culture of Dementia Care* (eds T. Kitwood & S. Benson), Hawker Publications, London.

Kitwood, T. (1997) *Dementia Reconsidered: The Person Comes First*, Open University Press, Buckingham.

Knapp, M., Thorgrimsen, L., Patel, A., Spector, A., Hallam, A., Woods, B., & Orrell, M. (2006) Cognitive stimulation therapy for people with dementia: cost-effectiveness analysis. *British Journal of Psychiatry,* **188**, 574–80.

Knopman, D., Rocca, W., Cha, R., Edland, S., & Kokmen, E. (2003) Survival study of vascular dementia in Rochester, Minnesota. *Archives of Neurology*, **60**(1), 85–90.

Koot, H. (2001) The study of quality of life: concepts and methods, in *Quality of Life in Child and Adolescent Illness* (eds H. Koot & J. Wallender), Taylor and Francis, New York.

Kukull, W., Larson, E., Reifler, B., Lampe, T., Yerby, M., & Hughes, J. (1990) The validity of three clinical diagnostic criteria for Alzheimer's disease. *Neurology*, **40**, 1364–9.

Lawton, M. (1994) Quality of Life in Alzheimer disease. *Alzheimer Disease and Associated Disorders*, **8**(3), 138–50.

Lawton, M. (1997) Assessing quality of life in Alzheimer's disease research. *Alzheimer Disease and Associated Disorders*, **11** (6), 91–9.

Lawton, M., & Brody, E. (1969) Assessment of older people: self-maintaining and instrumental activities of daily living. *Gerontologist*, **9**, 179–86.

Lawton, M., Van Haitsma, K., Perkinson, M., & Ruckdeschel, K. (1999) Observed affect and quality of life in dementia: further affirmations and problems. *Journal of Mental Health and Aging*, **5**, 69–82.

Livingston, G., Manela, M., & Katona, C. (1996) Depression and other psychiatric morbidity in carers of elderly people living at home. *British Medical Journal*, **312**, 153–6.

Logsdon, R., Gibbons, L., McCurry, S., & Teri, L. (2002) Assessing quality of life in older adults with cognitive impairment. *Psychosomatic Medicine*, **64**, 510–9.

Loiselle, L., & Dupuis, S. (2003) Let the music do the talking. *Aging, Health and Society: News and View*, **9**(1), 14–16.

Lowe, C., & Raynor, D. (2000) Intentional non-adherence in elderly patients: fact or fiction? *Pharmaceutical Journal*, **265** (Suppl.), R19.

Loy, C., & Schneider, L. (2004) Galantamine for Alzheimer's disease. *The Cochrane Database of Systematic Reviews* Issue 4, Art. No.: CD001747pub2. DOI: 10.1002/14651858CD001747pub2.

Lyness, J. (2004) End-of-life care. Issues relevant to the geriatric psychiatrist. *The American Journal of Geriatric Psychiatry*, **12**(5), 457–72.

MacDonald, A., & Dening, T. (2002) Dementia is being avoided in NHS and social care. *British Medical Journal*, **324**, 548.

McClendon, M., Smyth, K., & Neundorfer, M. (2004) Survival of persons with Alzheimer's disease: caregiver coping matters. *The Gerontologist*, **44**(4), 508–19.

McGowin, D. (1993) *Living in the Labyrinth: A Personal Journey through the Maze of Alzheimer's*, Mainsail Press, Cambridge.

Mack, J., & Whitehouse, P. (2001) Quality of life in dementia: state of the art – report of the international working group for the harmonization of dementia drug guidelines and the Alzheimer's society satellite meeting. *Alzheimer Disease and Associated Disorders*, **15**(2), 69–71.

McShane, R., Keene, J., Gedling, K., Fairburn, C., Jacoby, R., & Hope, T. (1997) Do neuroleptic drugs hasten cognitive decline in dementia? Prospective study with necropsy follow up. *British Medical Journal*, **314**, 266–70.

Marinker, M. (1997) From compliance to concordance: achieving shared goals in medicine taking. *British Medical Journal*, **314**, 747–8.

Max, W., Webber, P., & Fox, P. (1995) Alzheimer's disease the unpaid burden of caregiving. *Journal of Aging and Health*, **7**, 179–99.

Miesen, B. (1997) Awareness in dementia patients and family grieving: a practical perspective, in *Care-Giving in Dementia* (eds B. Miesen & G. Jones), Vol. 2, Routledge, London.

Misiorski, S. (2003) Pioneering culture change, in *Nursing Homes* [online], available: http://www.nursinghomesmagazine.com/Past_Issues.htm?ID=1518 [accessed 27 August 2006].

Morse, J., & Intrieri, R. (1997) 'Talk to me': patient communication in a long-term care facility. *Journal of Psychosocial Nursing*, **35**(5), 34–9.

Morton, I. (1997) Beyond validation, *in Mental Health for Elderly People* (eds I. Norman & S. Redfern), Churchill Livingstone, New York, pp. 371–93.

Myers, J. (2003) Coping with caregiving stress: a wellness-oriented, strengths-based approach for family counsellors. *The Family Journal: Counseling and Therapy for Couples and Families*, **12**(2), 153–61.

National Council for Palliative Care (2006) The palliative care needs for older people [online], available: www.ncpc.org.uk [accessed 4 June 2006].

National Institute for Health and Clinical Excellence (2001) *Guidance on the Use of Donepzil, Rivastigmine and Galantamine for the Treatment of Alzheimer's Disease*, London, http://www.nice.org.uk/page.aspx?o=14487.

National Institute for Health and Clinical Excellence (2005) *Appraisal Consultation Document; Donepzil, Rivastigmine, Galantamine and Memantine for the Treatment of Alzheimer's Disease*, London.

Neal, M., & Briggs, M. (2003) Validation therapy for dementia. *The Cochrane Database of Systematic Reviews*, Issue 3, Art. No.: CD001394. DOI:10.1002/14651858.CD001394.

Nolan, M., Grant, G., & Nolan, J. (1995) Busy doing nothing: activity and interaction levels amongst differing populations of elderly patients. *Journal of Advance Nursing*, **22**(3), 528–38.

Nolan, M., Ingram, P., & Watson, R. (2002) Working with family carers of people with dementia: 'negotiated' coping as an essential outcome. *Dementia*, **1**(1), 75–93.

Norris-Baker, L., Doll, G., Gray, L., & Kahl, J. (2003) Pioneering change. An illustrative guide to changing the culture of care in nursing homes with examples from the PEAK initiative [online], available: http://www.k-state.edu/peak/booklet/PEAKFIN1.PDF [accessed 27 August 2006].

Novack, D., Plumer, R., Smith, R., Ochtihill, H., Morrow, G., & Bennett, J. (1979) Changes in physicians' attitudes toward telling the cancer patient. *Journal of the American Medical Association*, **241**, 897–900.

Nursing and Midwifery Council (2004) The NMC code of professional conduct: standards for conduct, performance and ethics [online], available: http://www.nmc-uk.org/aFramedisplay.aspx?documentID=201 [accessed 16 September 2006].

Ory, M., Hoffman, R., Yee, J., Tennstedt, S., & Schulz, R. (1999) Prevalence and impact of caregiving: a detailed comparison between dementia and nondementia caregivers. *The Gerontologist*, **39**(2), 177–85.

O'Shea, E. (2003) Costs and consequences for the carers of people with dementia in Ireland. *Dementia*, **2**(2), 201–19.

Ostwald, S., Duggleby, W., & Hepburn, K. (2002) The stress of dementia: a view from the inside. *American Journal of Alzheimer's Disease and Other Dementias*, **17**(5), 303–12.

Overshott, R., & Burns, A. (2005) Treatment of dementia. *Journal of Neurology, Neurosurgery and Psychiatry*, **76**(Suppl. V), 53–9.

Overstall, P. (2005) How to recognise and treat depression in dementia. *Journal of Dementia Care*, **13**(3), 24–6.

Park, D., Hertzog, C., Leventhal, H., Morrell, R., Birchmore, D., Martin, M., & Bennett, J. (1999) Medication adherence in rheumatoid arthritis patients: older is wiser. *Journal of the American Geriatric Society*, **47**, 172–83.

Patrick, D., Starks, H., Cain, K., Uhlmann, R., & Pearlman, R. (1994) Measuring preferences for health states worse than death. *Medical Decision Making*, **14**, 9–18.

Perrin, T. (1997) Why are activities important? National Association for Providers of Activities for Older People [online], available: http://www.napaactivities.net/files/100011/Why%20activities%20are%20important%20Leaflet.doc [accessed 17 August 2006].

Perrin, T. (ed.) (2004) *The New Culture of Therapeutic Activity with Older People*, Speechmark Publishing Limited, Oxford.

Perrin, T. (2005) Let's stir up the outdated activity culture in care homes. *Journal of Dementia Care,* **13**(4), 26–7.

Perry, J., Galloway, S., Bottorf, J., & Nixon, S. (2005) Nurse–patient communication in dementia: improving the odds. *Journal of Gerontological Nursing,* **31**(4), 43–52.

Pinner, G. (2000) Truth-telling and the diagnosis of dementia. *British Journal of Psychiatry,* **176**, 514–5.

Powell, E. (1961) Water tower speech [online], available: www.mdx.ac.uk/www/study/ xpowell.htm [accessed 14 October 2005].

Pratt, R., & Wikinson, H. (2001) *Tell Me the Truth: The Effect of Being Told the Diagnosis of Dementia from the Perspective of the Person with Dementia,* Centre for Social Research on Dementia, University of Stirling.

Rabins, P. (1999) Developing scales to measure effective therapeutic interventions in quality of life in Alzheimer's disease. *Alzheimer Insights,* **5**(4), 7–9 [online], available: http://www.alzheimer-insights.com/pdf/5_4.pdf [accessed 25 July 2006].

Ready, R., & Ott, B. (2003) Quality of life measures for dementia. *Health and Quality of Life Outcomes,* **1**(11) [online], available: http://www.hqlo.com/content/1/1/11 [accessed 25 July 2006].

Ready, R., Ott, B., Grace, J., & Fernandez, I. (2002) The Cornell–Brown scale for quality of life in dementia. *Alzheimer Disease and Associated Disorders,* **16**, 109–15.

Reagan, R. (1994) [online], available: www.alz.org/media/newsreleases/ronaldreagan/ reaganletter.asp.

Report of the Metropolitan Commissioners in Lunacy to the Lord Chancellor (1844) [online], available: http://www.mdx.ac.uk/www/study/4_09.htm [accessed 10 October 2005].

Rollin, H. (2003) Psychiatry in Britain one hundred years ago. *British Journal of Psychiatry,* **183**, 292–8.

Royal College of Psychiatrists (2001) *Mental Illness: Stigmatisation and Discrimination within the Medical Profession,* Council Report CR91, Royal College of Psychiatrists, Royal College of Physicians, London.

Royal College of Psychiatrists (2006) *Changing Minds: Every Family in the Land* [online], available: http://www.rcpsych.ac.uk/campaigns/changingminds. aspx [30 October 2006].

Royal College of Psychiatrists (2005) *Forgetful but not Forgotten: Assessment and Aspects of Treatment of People with Dementia by a Specialist Old Age Psychiatry Service,* Royal College of Psychiatrists, London.

Royal College of Psychiatrists Faculty for the Psychiatry of Old Age (2004) *Atypical Antipsychotics and Behavioural and Psychiatric Symptoms of Dementia, Prescribing Update for Old Age Psychiatrists,* [online], available: http://www.rcpsych.ac.uk/ college/faculty/oap/BPSD.pdf [accessed 18 February 2005].

Ruddock, R. (1969) *Roles and Relationships,* Routledge and Kegan Paul, London.

Sabat, S. (2002) Surviving manifestations of selfhood in Alzheimer's disease. *Dementia,* **1**(1), 25–36.

Sachs, G., Shega, M., & Cox-Hayley, D. (2004) Barriers to excellent end-of-life care for patients with dementia. *Journal of General Internal Medicine,* **19**, 1057–63.

Schulz, R., & Beach, S. (1999) Caregiving as a risk factor for mortality: the caregiver health effects study. *Journal of the American Medical Association,* **282**, 2215–9.

Schulz, R., O'Brien, A., Bookwala, J., & Fleissner, K. (1995) Pyschiatric and physical morbidity effects of dementia caregiving: prevalence, correlates, and causes. *The Gerontologist,* **35**(6), 771–91.

Setterlund, D. (1998) Dementia care staff and family carers: their relationships in the context of care. *Australasian Journal on Ageing*, **17**(3), 135–9.

Sheard, D. (2004) Person centred care: the emperor's new clothes? *Journal of Dementia Care*, **12**(2), 22–5.

Sheldon, B. (1994) Communicating with Alzheimer's patients. *Journal of Gerontological Nursing*, **20**(10), 51–3.

Shuster, J. (2006) Caring when we cannot cure: research in geriatric palliative care [online], available: http://cmha.ua.edu/Caring%20When%20We%20Cannon%20Cure-Research%20in%20Geratric%20Palliative%20Care.ppt#269,18,Goals%20of%20Palliative%20Care [accessed 27 May 2006].

Signpost (2006) [online], available: http://www.signpostjournal.co.uk/welcome.htm [accessed 15 September 2006].

Small, J., & Perry, J. (2005) Do you remember? How caregivers question their spouses who have Alzheimer's disease and the impact on communication. *Journal of Speech, Language, and Hearing Research*, **48**, 125–36.

Smith Henderson, C. (1998) *Partial View. An Alzheimer's Journal.* Southern Methodist University Press, Dallas.

Spector, A., Orrell, M., Davies, S., & Woods, B. (2000) Reality orientation for dementia. *The Cochrane Database of Systematic Reviews*, Issue 3, Art. No.: CD001119. DOI: 10.1002/14651858.CD001119.

Spector, A., Thorgrimsen, L., Woods, B., Royan, L., Davies, S., Butterworth, M., & Orrell, M. (2003) Efficacy of an evidence-based cognitive stimulation therapy programme for people with dementia: randomised controlled trial. *British Journal of Psychiatry*, **183**, 248–54.

Stanton, L., & Coetzee, R. (2004) Down's syndrome and dementia. *Advances in Psychiatric Treatment*, **10**, 50–8.

Stokes, G. (2000) *Challenging Behaviour in Dementia: A Person Centred Approach*, Winslow Press, Bicester.

Sullivan, R., Menapace, L., & White, R. (2001) Truth-telling and patient diagnoses. *Journal of Medical Ethics*, **27**, 192–7.

Svanström, R., & Dahlberg, K. (2004) Living with dementia yields a heteronomous and lost existence. *Western Journal of Nursing Research*, **26**(6), 671–87.

Tappen, R.M., Williams, C., Fishman, S., & Touhy, T. (1999) Persistance of self in advanced Alzheimer's disease. *Image Journal of Nursing Scholar*, **31**(2), 121–5.

Tarlow, B., Wisniewski, S., Belle, S., Rubert, M., Ory, M., & Gallagher-Thompson, D. (2004) Positive aspects of caregiving: contributions of the REACH project to the development of new measures for Alzheimer's caregiving. *Research on Aging*, **26**(4), 429–53.

Tester, S., Hubbard, G., Downs, M., MacDonald, C., & Murphy, J. (2003) Exploring perceptions of quality of life of frail older people during and after their transition to institutional care, in *Research Findings* [online], available: http://www.esrc.ac.uk/ESRCInfoCentre/Plain_English_Summaries/LLH/index149.aspx?ComponentId=9591&SourcePageId=11772 [accessed 18 July 2006].

The Economist Intelligence Unit's Quality-of-Life Index (2005) [online], available: http://www.economist.com/media/pdf/QUALITY_OF_LIFE.pdf [accessed 17 July 2006].

Thornicroft, G., & Tansella, M. (2003) *What are the arguments for community-based mental health care?*. WHO Health Evidence Network [online], available: www.who.dk/eprise/main/WHO/Progs/HEN/Syntheses/mentalhealth/20030822_1 [accessed 25 October 2005].

Tombs, S. (1997) Design for dementia: six conference papers. Dementia Services Development Centre, University of Stirling [online], available: http://www.dementia.stir.ac.uk/pdf/Design.pdf [accessed 18 August 2006].

Treloar, A., Beck, S., & Paton, C. (2001) Administering medicines to patients with dementia and other organic syndromes. *Advances in Psychiatric Treatment*, **7**, 444–52.

Trick, L., & Obcarskas, S. (1968) *Understanding Mental Illness and Its Nursing*, Pitman Medical Publishing Company Limited, London.

United Kingdom Central Council for Nursing, Midwifery and Health Visiting (1986) *Project 2000 – A New Preparation for Practice*, UKCC, London.

Verdantam, S. (2004) Reagan's experience alters outlook for Alzheimer's patients. *The Washington Post,* **10**, June 14.

Vig, E., Davenport, N., & Pearlman, R. (2002) Good deaths, bad deaths, and preferences for the end of life: a qualitative study of geriatric outpatients. *Journal of the American Geriatric Society,* **50**(9), 1541–8.

Vink, A., Birks, J., Bruinsma, M., & Scholten, R. (2003) Music therapy for people with dementia. *The Cochrane Database of Systematic Reviews*, Issue 4, Art. No.: CD003477. DOI: 10.1002/14651858.CD003477pub2.

Volicer, L. (2005) End-of-life care for people with dementia in residential care settings. Executive summary [online], available: http://www.alz.org/Health/Care/endoflifelitreview.pdf [accessed 25 March 2006].

Walker, A. (1995) Integrating the family in the mixed economy of care, in *The Future of Family Care for Older People* (eds I. allen & E. Perkins), HMSO, London.

Wang, P., Schneeweiss, S., Avorn, J., Fischer, M., Mogun, H., Soloman, D., & Brookhart, M. (2005) Risk of death in elderly users of conventional vs. atypical antipsychotic medications. *The New England Journal of Medicine*, **353**(22), 2335–41.

Ward, R., Vass, A., Aggarwal, N., Garfield, C., Cybyk, B., & Minardi, H. (2002) Dementia, communication and care: 1. Expanding our understanding. *Journal of Dementia Care*, **10**(5), 33–6.

Ward, R., Vass, A., Aggarwal, N., Garfield, C., & Cybyk, B. (2005) What is dementia care? 1. Dementia is communication. *Journal of Dementia Care,* **13**(6), 16–19.

Ward, R., Vass, A., Aggarwal, N., Garfield, C., & Cybyk, B. (2006) What is dementia care? 2. An invisible workload. *Journal of Dementia Care,* **14**(1), 28–30.

Warner, J., Butler, R., & Wuntakal, B. (2005) Dementia [online], available: http://www.clinicalevidence.com/ceweb/conditions/meh/1001/1001_contribdetails.jsp.

Weiner, M., Martin-Cook, K., Svetlik, D., Saine, K., Foster, B., & Fontaine, C. (2000) The quality of life in late-stage dementia (QUALID) scale. *Journal of the American Medical Directors Association,* **1**, 114–16.

Westbury, J. (2003) Why do older people not always take their medication? *The Pharmaceutical Journal*, **271**, 503–4.

Wilkinson, H. (2002) Including people with dementia in research: methods and motivations, in *The Perspective of People with Dementia: Research Methods and Motivations* (ed. H. Wilkinson), Jessica Kingsley, London.

World Health Organization (1992) *International Classification of Diseases*, 10th edn, World Health Organization, Geneva.

World Health Organization (2001) Mental health problems: the undefined and hidden burden, Fact Sheet No. 218 [online], available: http://www.who.int/mediacentre/factsheets/fs218/en/print.html [accessed 23 March 2005].

World Health Organization (2004a) Health evidence network. *What is the Effectiveness of Old-Age Mental Health Services?* [online], available: www.euro.who.int/eprise/main/WHO/Progs/HEN/Syntheses/mentalservice/20040720_2 [accessed 21 February 2006].

World Health Organization (2004b) *Better Palliative Care for Older People* (eds E. Davies & I. Higginson) [online], available: http://www.euro.who.int/document/E82933pdf [accessed 30 May 2006].

Yale, R. (1995) *Developing Support Groups for Individuals with Early-Stage Alzheimer's Disease. Planning, Implementation and Evaluation*, Health Professions Press, Baltimore.

Zimmerman, S., Williams, C., Reed, P., Boustani, M., Preisser, J., Heck, E., & Sloane, P. (2005) Attitudes, stress and satisfaction of staff who care for residents with dementia. *The Gerontologist*, **45** (Suppl. 1), 96–105.

Index

abuse 1, 45, 155, 177
  in advanced dementia 157–62
  incidence 159
  medication 147
Academy of Molecular Imaging 23
acceptance coping 86
acetylcholinesterase 26–7
acetylcholinesterase inhibitors 7, 9, 11, 26,
    135, 147, 148–50
activities of daily living (ADL) 128,
    130
activity, meaningful 123–5
advance directive 127, 163, 164, 165
advance statement 163, 164, 165
advanced dementia 156–7
  abuse in 157–62
ageism 16
aggression 11, 109, 110, 113, 145
alcohol abuse 4, 5
Alzheimer Scotland 14
Alzheimer's Association of America 23
Alzheimer's Australia 23
Alzheimer's disease 2, 6–7, 11
  disclosure 54, 57
  drug treatment 57, 147
  genetics of 6
  identification 38
  insight in 75
  survival time 155
Alzheimer's Disease International 26, 90
Alzheimer's Society 13, 14, 21, 25–6, 27,
    63, 147, 176, 184, 186
  Food for Thought project 26
anger 1, 77, 78
antibiotics 166–7
antidepressant medication 79
antipsychotic medication 112, 145–8
anxiety 40, 54, 79, 107
apathy 79, 80
aphasia 156
appetite, changes in 79
assessment 113
asylums 15, 28, 31, 32, 41
Australia, dementia burden in 14

behavioural and psychological symptoms of
    dementia (BPSD) 145, 146–7
behavioural therapy 37
benzodiazepines 151
Biography (life history) 43, 46
bipolar disorder 40, 112, 145
blame 18
Blyton, Enid 22
boredom 77–8, 110
brain tumours 4
Briggs report 33
British Geriatric Society 157, 160
Bronson, Charles 22
burden 14, 80, 84, 91
burn-out 86, 106

cardiopulmonary resuscitation 166
carers
  burden to 86
  challenging behaviour and 113–14
  depression and anxiety in 85
  fatigue in 85
  impact on 84–8
  psychiatric morbidity in 85
Carey, Dr Nicholas 25
caring relationship 41, 44, 45–7
challenging behaviour 1, 93, 145, 180
  in advanced dementia 156
  as communication 108–12
  resolving 112–14
children living with dementia 88–90
chlorpromazine 28, 145
clinical governance 31
cognitive stimulation therapy (CST) 68,
    124
communication 71, 82, 93–116, 180
  to children 90
  content of 99
  environment and 98, 101
  impact of dementia on 95–8
  importance of 94–5
  organisational barriers to 98–100
  quality of life and 131–2
  research difficulties 101–4

Please remember that this is a library book,
and that it belongs only temporarily to each
person who uses it. Be considerate. Do
not write in this, or any, library book.